D0743765

PEOPLE-CENTRED
HEALTH PROMOTION

This book is dedicated
to the memory of
Joan Atkinson
and
Sam Albert
two truly
"people-centred" people!

PEOPLE-CENTRED HEALTH PROMOTION

John Raeburn
and
Irving Rootman

JOHN WILEY & SONS

Chichester · New York · Weinheim · Brisbane · Singapore · Toronto

Copyright © 1998 by John Wiley & Sons Ltd,
Baffins Lane, Chichester,
West Sussex PO19 1UD, England

National   01243 779777
International (+44) 1243 779777
e-mail (for orders and customer service enquiries): cs-books@wiley.co.uk
Visit our Home Page on http://www.wiley.co.uk
or http://www.wiley.com

All Rights Reserved. No part of this book may be reproduced, stored in a retrieval system, or
transmitted, in any form or by any means, electronic, mechanical, photocopying, recording,
scanning or otherwise, except under the terms of the Copyright, Designs and Patents Act 1988
or under the terms of a licence issued by the Copyright Licensing Agency, 90 Tottenham Court
Road, London, UK W1P 9HE, without the permission in writing of the publisher.

Other Wiley Editorial Offices

John Wiley & Sons, Inc., 605 Third Avenue,
New York, NY 10158-0012, USA

WILEY-VCH Verlag GmbH, Pappelallee 3,
D-69469 Weinheim, Germany

Jacaranda Wiley Ltd, 33 Park Road, Milton,
Queensland 4064, Australia

John Wiley & Sons (Asia) Pte Ltd, 2 Clementi Loop #02-01,
Jin Xing Distripark, Singapore 129809

John Wiley & Sons (Canada) Ltd, 22 Worcester Road,
Rexdale, Ontario M9W 1LI, Canada

Library of Congress Cataloging-in-Publication Data

Raeburn, John (John Maxwell)
    People-centred health promotion / John Raeburn and Irving Rootman.
    p.   cm.
    Includes bibliographical references and index.
    ISBN 0-471-97791-8 (hardbound). — ISBN 0-471-97137-5 (pbk.)
    1. Health promotion.   I. Rootman, I.   II. Title.
    RA427.8.R34   1997
    613—dc21   97–22463
                                                                   CIP

British Library Cataloguing in Publication Data

A catalogue record for this book is available from the British Library

ISBN 0-471-97791-8 (cased)
ISBN 0-471-97137-5 (paper)

Typeset in 10/12pt Palatino from the author's disks by by Dorwyn Ltd, Rowlands Castle,
Hants.
Printed and bound in Great Britain by Bookcraft (Bath) Ltd, Midsomer Norton, Somerset
This book is printed on acid-free paper responsibly manufactured from sustainable
forestation, for which at least two trees are planted for each one used for paper production.

CONTENTS

Foreword vii
Preface ix
Acknowledgements xi

Part I   Introduction

1   People-Centred Health Promotion: What is it?   3

2   People-Centred Health Promotion: The key essentials 16

3   Placing PCHP in the theoretical and political spectrum 45

Part II   Basic concepts, issues and approach

4   The overall aim of PCHP: Health and well-being in a quality
    of life context 53

5   Empowerment 64

6   Community development 80

7   Cultural dimensions 98

8   Spiritual dimensions 111

Part III   The practice of PCHP

9   Applying PCHP principles: General considerations and
    introduction to the People System 129

10   The People System: A general guide 138

11   The People System: Outcome evaluation 152

12   Case studies I: Community Push and the Birkdale–Beachhaven
     Community Project 167

13   Case studies II: Superhealth 182

14   Case studies III: The North Shore Community Health Network
     and the Other Way Project 196

15   Towards a PCHP society 214

References 224
Index 229

FOREWORD

From Preface to Postscript, this book engages the reader in an intellectually challenging and socially compelling enterprise. The challenge is the work of improving the health of populations by means other than medical and technological. The enterprise is called health promotion; the methods of choice are people-centred. The authors are known internationally for their leadership in forging a definition of this field and these methods.

The authors' first task was to trace the modern (and post-modern) history of health promotion. The point from whence to begin that story can be debated among academic and professional disciplines who can cite elements of latter-day health promotion in their writings of decades ago. Parts of people-centered health promotion appeared even centuries ago, if one interprets Egyptian, Babylonian, Biblical, ancient Chinese, Koranic, Hindu, Buddhist, Greek and Roman texts as more than philosophical or religious admonitions. Professors Raeburn and Rootman pick up these threads in 1974, when Marc Lalonde, then Minister of Health for Canada, introduced health promotion as a "New perspective on the Health of Canadians."

Central to the Lalonde Report, and subsequent governmental initiatives in Canada, the United States, New Zealand, Australia, the United Kingdom, some Scandinavian countries, and the Netherlands, was the neglected importance of lifestyle as a determinant of health. This emphasis on lifestyle devolved in a conservative era to an excessively focused emphasis on self-control and specific behavioural risk factors. Enlightened health promotion practitioners and writers continued to develop a more robust concept of lifestyle with intellectual and research roots in sociology and anthropology. The more robust notion was that lifestyle was not just what people could do for themselves if they exercised greater self-control and discipline in their health-directed behaviour. It also encompassed what communities—people in their extended families, workplaces, ethnic attachments, schools and other institutions making up the social milieu—can do to support each other in developing and maintaining more healthful cultures and social structures.

The practitioners of health promotion found themselves during this era, and still do, in a withering crossfire between the more-rigorous-than-thou rhetoric from the radically reductionist, scientific wing of health promotion on one side and the more-equitable-than-thou rhetoric of the politically correct wing on the other. Raeburn and Rootman have established a beachhead where people live.

Between the victim blamers on one side and the system blamers on the other, a people-based approach to health promotion plants its feet on a community "centre of gravity" (as Raeburn and I called it in an earlier attempt to position health promotion). Between the misplaced precision of micro-interventionists and the sometimes misplaced policies of the macro-interventionists lies a level of intervention in which Raeburn and Rootman urge attention to the close-to-home social fabric of the people affected by interventions. They suggest methods of understanding, consulting, working with and, ultimately, safeguarding the empowerment of those who would benefit from health promotion. This people-centred approach to health promotion pulls us back to our commitment to healthy people after some lost energy on trying to anthropomorphize healthy schools, healthy public policy, and healthy workplaces. It builds on the energy in those movements but with a reminder that it is the health of people for which society ultimately will hold health promotion accountable.

This book does not pretend to be an academic reference or textbook in the usual sense. It is a book about the heart of health promotion; it pleads for staying in touch with the people, communities and empowerment perspectives of health promotion. It is a counterweight, if not an antidote, to the sometimes overworked parts of the Ottawa Charter that emphasized a potentially faceless policy and macro-systems approach to health promotion. One might view this as a third wave in the evolution of health promotion from its behavioural roots through the Ottawa Charter era which tried to focus away from individual behaviour and onto the broadest social and economic environments that condition the lifestyles of whole populations. One might, alternatively, regard this as taming the pendulum swings from those widely polar extremes to a balancing or converging of both on the community cultural factors that are most meaningful to people.

The book's emphasis on culture also admits a greater emphasis on the spiritual dimensions of health, the soul of health, than most prevailing secular models and efforts in health promotion have allowed themselves. The book is full of idealism, but the final part with its People System and its application, and with case studies, shows how to translate the idealism into real projects. The last chapter presents a vision for a society built on health promotion values.

Lawrence W. Green
University of British Columbia

PREFACE

This book is a collaborative undertaking by two people from different countries and with different backgrounds. One of us, John Raeburn, is a New Zealander and a psychologist who teaches behavioural science and health promotion to medical and health science students, and who has worked in a hands-on way in community development and community health promotion settings for many years. The other, Irving Rootman, is a Canadian and a sociologist, who before his present appointment as Director of the Health Promotion Centre of the University of Toronto worked for many years in the Federal Government Health Promotion Directorate as a researcher and manager.

The two of us met in 1986, in the Health Promotion Directorate in Ottawa, where John spent a year's sabbatical and Irving was Director of Research. These were the heady days leading up to the international conference that produced the Ottawa Charter, and the Directorate was humming with new ideas and planning for new policy directions. We both attended the Ottawa conference, John as a New Zealand delegate, and Irving as one of the hosts.

It was during 1986 that we found we worked well together, sparking ideas off each other and enjoying the process greatly. This resulted in our collaborating on a number of theoretical and other writings. In 1993, we met in Toronto, and decided to do this book together.

One of the major themes that drives the work and outlook of both of us is the importance of *people* in health promotion. We are both "people people", so to speak, and this belief in and liking for people is what underlies this book.

It has not always been easy trying to write a book in different countries, and no amount of faxes or e-mail messages can substitute for the liveliness of face-to-face discussion. But we hope some of the spirit of enjoyment and excitement that switch us on about the eternally fascinating area of health promotion is communicated to you, the reader, in these pages. We feel the breadth of perspective and experience we can bring to this work because of our different locations and backgrounds adds a dimension that neither of us could have achieved alone.

So who is this book for, and what is it trying to do? We see the audience as being our students, colleagues, and others like them. It is not intended to be a formal textbook, so much as a structure around which a course in health promotion could be built. We do not attempt to dot all the i's and cross all the t's. Rather, we assume a relatively mature audience whom we would like to stimulate with ideas for discussion, who can then do further study independently, and who will draw their own conclusions.

The style is deliberately light, and, we hope, easy to read. But the message is deeply felt. As the 21st century approaches, the juggernauts of technology, international finance, population growth, conflict and poverty show no sign of abating. The potential for facelessness, alienation and violence is even more powerful now than it was when these factors were first identified by sociologists a century ago as products of the industrial revolution. The people-centred health promotion presented in this book argues for a set of human values and a "true democracy" which are seen as buffers against some of the "mega-trends" that currently seem to have us in their grip. We do not delude ourselves that this sort of approach will reverse these trends. But it could help to make life more tolerable, healthy and happy in the face of a future that may otherwise be a very unhealthy one. We hope you will share this view.

John Raeburn
Irving Rootman

ACKNOWLEDGEMENTS

There are many people who have contributed to this book, and to the projects and thinking that lie behind it.

They are too numerous to mention here, but we thank you all.

There is just one person we would like to acknowledge by name, and that is Denise Reynolds, whose indefatigable labour on many versions of the manuscript, quality of work, and unfailing good cheer and wisdom make her a very special person.

Thank you, Denise.

The authors are very grateful to all the copyright holders who have given them permission to reproduce previously published material in this volume:

Chapter 5: On pages 70–73, from Kieffer, C. (1984) Citizen empowerment: A developmental perspective. *Prevention in Human Services*, **3**, 9–36. Reproduced by permission of The Haworth Press, Inc., New York. On pages 74–76, from Labonte, R. (1993) Health promotion and empowerment: Practice frameworks. *Issues in Health Promotion*, vol. III: Toronto: Centre for Health Promotion/ParticipACTION. Reproduced by permission. On pages 65–67, from Lord, J. and Farlow, D. M. (1990) A study of personal empowerment: Implications for health promotion. Originally published in *Health Promotion (Canada)*, **29**, 2–8. On pages 67–69, from Rappaport, J. (1981) In praise of paradox: A social policy of empowerment over prevention. *American Journal of Community Psychology*, **9**, 1–25. Reproduced by permission of Plenum Publishing Corp., New York.

Chapter 6: On pages 96–97, from Boyte, H. C. (1989) People power transforms a St Louis housing project. *Utne Reader*, **34**, 46–47. Originally published in Occasional Papers (Jan. 1989), Community Renewal Society, Chicago. On pages 86–87, from Breckon, D. J., Harvey, J. R. and Lancaster, R. B. (1985) *Community Health Education*. Rockville, MD: Aspen. Reproduced by permission. On pages 93–95, from Durning, A. B. (1989) Grass roots groups are our best hope for global prosperity and ecology. *Utne Reader*, **34**, 40–49. Copyright 1989 *World Watch Magazine*. Reproduced by permission of World

Watch Institute. On pages 87–92, from Minkler, M. (1990) Improving health through community organization. In K. Glanze, F. M. Lewis and B. K. Rimer (Eds), *Health Behavior and Health Education*, pp. 257-287. San Francisco, CA: Jossey-Bass. Copyright 1990 Jossey-Bass, Inc., Publishers. Reproduced by permission of Jossey-Bass/Pfeiffer, Simon & Schuster International and Business & Professional Group. On pages 81–83, from Shirley, I. (Ed.) (1982) *Development Tracks: The Theory and Practice of Community Development*. Palmerston North: Dunmore Press. Reproduced by permission of Dunmore Press.

Chapter 7: On pages 101–104, from Kinloch, P. (1985) *Talking Health but Doing Sickness: Studies in Samoan Health*. Wellington: Victoria University Press. Reproduced by permission. On pages 107–108, from Rangihau, J. (1992) Being Maori. In M. King (Ed.), *Te Ao Hurihuri: Aspects of Maoritanga*. Auckland: Reed. Copyright 1992 John Rangihau. Reproduced by permission. On pages 104–105, from Walker, R. (1982) Development from below: Institutional transformation in a plural society. In I. Shirley (Ed.), *Development Tracks: The Theory and Practice of Community Development*. Palmerston North: Dunmore Press. Reproduced by permission of Dunmore Press.

Chapters 7 & 8: On pages 103 and 117, from Ngan-Woo, F. (1990) *Faasamoa: The World of Samoans*, Auckland: Office of the Race Relations Conciliator.

Chapter 8: On pages 121–124, from Brandon, D. (1976) *Zen in the Art of Helping*. London: Routledge & Kegan-Paul. On pages 120–121, from Claxton, G. (1986) *Beyond Therapy: The Impact of Eastern Religions on Psychological Theory and Practice*. London: Wisdom. Reprinted by Prism Press. On pages 124–125, from Nhat Hanh, T. (1987) *Being Peace*. Berkeley, CA: Parallax Press. Reproduced by permission of Parallax Press.

I

INTRODUCTION

In Part I, we look at the concept of People-Centred Health Promotion (PCHP). We view PCHP as perhaps representing a "third wave" in health promotion, following the lifestyle and social model eras. Our concerns arise especially from the fact that much health promotion today seems to take a somewhat "depersonalized" view, relying as it does on statistics, a population perspective and a traditional social science paradigm. Our contention is that health promotion, above all other endeavours, is an intensely personal and human area, and should begin from a perspective of people's experience, in the context of their everyday community lives.

There are three chapters in Part I. Chapter 1 looks at the history of health promotion, and the development of health promotion as a concept. PCHP is briefly introduced. In Chapter 2, PCHP is considered in some detail, with the aid of the mnemonic PEOPLE, which stands for *P*eople-centredness, *Em*powerment, *O*rganizational and community development, *P*articipation, *L*ife quality and *E*valuation. At the core of the approach we are advocating are the two concepts of empowerment and community development. Chapter 3 places PCHP in its academic and political context. Since health promotion covers a variety of disciplines and has a strong political and social justice feel about it, it is important to know where we are coming from when we adopt a stance in the area.

1

PEOPLE-CENTRED HEALTH PROMOTION
What is it?

This book is about "people-centred health promotion" (PCHP). To use such a term at all implies that there are varieties of health promotion that are not people-centred, or at least not as people-centred as they could be. So first we will take an overview of health promotion as a field, and see where its "people" aspects are deficient. Then we will go on to look at the key characteristics of a PCHP.

WHAT IS HEALTH PROMOTION?
The Beginnings of the Modern Era

Most people date the beginning of the modern era of health promotion from the "Lalonde Report", a Canadian government document published in 1974 under the name of Marc Lalonde, the then Minister of National Health and Welfare (Lalonde, 1974).

It is worth looking for a moment at the Lalonde Report, because just about everything that has happened in health promotion since then has either arisen directly out of its philosophy and recommendations, or been a reaction to it.

The Lalonde Report presented convincing statistics showing that, in spite of the fact that in 1971 Canada was spending 7.1% of its GNP on health, and that this figure was growing, Canadians' health was not improving. The health problems of particular concern were the "diseases of affluence" (as distinct from the infectious diseases), such as heart disease, cancer, drug and alcohol addiction, sexually transmitted diseases, and respiratory disease associated with smoking and pollution, as well as injuries arising from road accidents. Most of the deaths from these causes (and they accounted for over

70% of all deaths) were regarded as premature (before the age of 70), involving in a given year an unnecessary loss of some 800 000 years of life in a population of 20 million. More, it was asserted that these premature illnesses and deaths were, in the main, the product of "lifestyle", which in the Lalonde Report mainly meant the areas of drug and alcohol abuse, smoking, fitness and recreation, nutrition and sexual behaviour. It was argued, since these behaviours are all potentially modifiable, the cost and incidence of the diseases of affluence and their attendant premature mortality could be reduced.

What was especially radical about the Lalonde Report was its assertion that positive changes in the health state of affairs were not going to be brought about by going down the same publicly funded health track as before. Until that time, it was pointed out, most tax money had gone into "health services"—that is, services such as hospitals and clinics set up to attend to those who are *sick*. The report argued for a "new perspective", one which would direct public money towards, amongst other things, a "health promotion strategy". This, as far as we know, was the first time a government had made a major statement of this nature, and one only has to be aware of the power of the health service establishment to realize that such an expression of intention to direct funds away from existing services into "health promotion" would be a challenging exercise for any government. Nevertheless, the arguments were so compelling, and the methods to do something about it so seemingly straightforward, that by 1978, the Canadian government had set up in Ottawa a new Health Promotion Directorate, part of its Federal Department of Health and Welfare, with about a hundred staff—the first such venture in the world. (Most Western countries now have some comparable agency.)

There is no doubt that the concept for which the Lalonde Report will always be remembered is that of "lifestyle", which it introduced into the health arena. Interestingly enough, this concept was embedded in a larger entity called the "Health Field Concept", which "envisages that the health field can be broken up into four broad elements: Human Biology, Environment, Lifestyle and Health Care Organization" (p. 31). However, the human mind being what it is, the simplest and most exciting concept was abstracted from this, and "lifestyle" became the dominant preoccupation of health promotion for the next decade or so.

At the time of the Lalonde Report, it is probably true to say that the professional groupings with the most expertise in health behaviour and its modification were health educators and psychologists. Everyone conceded that for lifestyle change to take place in the community, "education" was needed. That is, people needed to know the facts related to the links between behaviour and health (e.g. that smoking causes heart disease and lung cancer), and also needed to know what could be done to improve their health.

This required knowledge, persuasion and education. Hence, "health education" was one clearly relevant discipline. However, health behaviour is notoriously hard to change, and this raised the issue of how best to modify behaviour, which is in the province of psychology.

In the 1970s, psychology courses were (and still are) among the most popular available at most North American universities. Psychologists are also probably the most powerful "health" group outside medicine and paramedical professions such as nursing. One of the chief topics of interest to psychologists at that time was behaviour modification. So it was natural that the methods of psychology should be looked at to bring about the desired changes in people.

All these trends were reinforced by another set of historical events, this time coming from the USA. Because of the size, wealth and influence of that country, things American tend to have a huge impact on us in the West. In the 1970s the health promotion area was no exception. The American events of significance at this time were the publication of a government document called *Healthy people: The Surgeon General's report on health promotion and disease prevention* (Surgeon General, 1979), and the subsequent setting of 226 quantified prevention and health promotion "Objectives for the Nation" to be achieved by the year 1990. What we had in the USA was a version of health promotion that was ideologically very similar to Canada's, but which was on a more ambitious scale, and more explicitly attuned to goals and behaviour modification. These goals have now been updated and the timetable has been extended to the year 2000, so that this approach has been cemented in on a grand scale to the end of the century, with all or most states agreeing to be part of the Objectives for the Nation exercise. While America still seems to be going down that track, at least some of the rest of the world, including Canada, have taken a different direction—of which more shortly.

The Ottawa Charter and the "New Direction"

The Canadian and American moves had awakened a new consciousness in the world. At least in theory, public resources in the health field were no longer to be exclusively the province of biomedicine and the curative health services. Now other players could enter the fray. At first, these were mainly health educators and psychologists. But other professions and academic disciplines were also starting to stake their claim.

As is often the case when academic and professional groups are in competition, attempts were made to discredit the theoretical and practice base of the other groups. It was not long before the lifestyle model of health promotion came under attack. From a theoretical point of view, this attack came from two main directions.

One of these had to do with "victim blaming". The lifestyle model tended to lead to statements like: "Your lung cancer is caused by smoking. If you didn't smoke, you wouldn't have lung cancer. Therefore you are to blame for your lung cancer". However, if we go beyond the surface of most people's lives, we find that decisions to smoke, drink too much, engage in unsafe sex, etc. are not simply matters of rational choice, but are embedded in complex social situations. For example, what a person eats is closely related to income, education, upbringing, culture, and so on. So to "blame" someone for a life situation that is often beyond their control—and often the more miserable it is, the more "unhealthy" behaviours seem to exist—was simply not fair.

The second area of criticism related to social class issues. As had been known for a long time, there is a "gradient" of ill health and mortality closely related to one's position in the social order. That is, the lower one is down the social scale, the poorer one's health. What this shows is similar to the conclusion drawn from the victim-blaming critique—that the forces determining health status are not just "lifestyle" in the abstract, but are the product of a complex array of social factors. Indeed, although the effects of ill health may be via lifestyle (lower class people, for example, smoke more), lifestyle in turn is determined by all sorts of cultural, self-esteem, power, financial, stress, and other such considerations. In addition, the physical environment, pollution, city design, accommodation, water supplies, noise, a state of war, nuclear fallout, political instability, unemployment, and many other such factors can all be shown to be directly related to health status. Collectively, these observations all lend weight to what has become known as the "social model" of health, the main opposition stance to a lifestyle model in the health promotion area.

Perhaps the strongest protagonist of the social model has been the World Health Organization (WHO), and it was the WHO who largely engineered the Ottawa Charter for Health Promotion, certainly the single most influential document on the international health promotion scene (Ottawa Charter, 1986). It is notable that the Ottawa Charter mentions the term "lifestyle" only once, and then to dismiss it as somewhat inadequate. ("Health promotion . . . goes beyond healthy life-styles to well-being.") Rather, we are told that health is "a positive concept emphasizing social and personal resources, as well as physical capacities", and that the prerequisites for health are not so much lifestyle as "peace, shelter, education, food, income, a stable ecosystem, sustainable resources, social justice and equity". In this context, health promotion is not a matter of changing lifestyle, but "of enabling people to increase control over, and to improve, their health". However, what probably appeals to people most about the Ottawa Charter is its breaking down of the concerns of health promotion into five areas on which planning for action can be based. These five action streams of the Ottawa

Charter are: build public policy; create supportive environments; strengthen community action; develop personal skills; and reorient health services. As can be seen, the Ottawa Charter is both a philosophical and a practical document, although in practice many health promotion workers have found it difficult to use the Charter in any but the most general terms.

What also tended to happen along with throwing out the lifestyle concept was a playing down of the role of the "individual" as an agent in her or his own health promotion. Many of the people most influential in criticizing the earlier versions of health promotion were social scientists who preferred to operate in broad terms of "society", "structures", "policy", "populations", and the like, rather than in terms of the individual.

Yet what individual people *do*—how they think, behave, act, support each other, and so on—*does* influence health, and the social forces outlined in the Ottawa Charter have their impact on populations through the heads, bodies and behaviour of individuals in their everyday, real-life, community situations.

To sum up, then, the history of health promotion since the 1970s has been one of an area swaying from one ideological stance to another, with quite fundamentally different views being expressed about the essential nature of the enterprise. We also suspect that in some countries there is little political will to support health promotion anyway in spite of the passions it engenders in its advocates. Until recently, the prevailing health promotion ideology internationally appears to have been the social model, although our feeling is that maybe not too many of those actually working in the field have taken this to their hearts. In this book, we would like us to move beyond the lifestyle versus social model debate, and return to a health promotion that is vitally concerned with *people*. This is not to say that populations, policy, and so on are not important—they *are* extremely important. But we believe that the analysis of such factors should serve the *real* purpose of health promotion, which is (in our view) a better life and better health and well-being for everyone, especially those who tend to get neglected.

PEOPLE-CENTRED HEALTH PROMOTION

In general terms, there tend to be two major groups of people working in health promotion—those who interact directly with people, and those who make policy. The agendas that drive these two groups are often quite different.

Those who work directly with people tend to be further down the occupational scale—nurses, community workers, health educators, agency workers, volunteers, and so on. Those who work with policy tend to be in positions of greater power, and often seem to have the backing of academics.

The people-workers tend to understand people and community process. The policy-makers understand statistics, economic factors, politics, and so on.

There is no doubt that most people who work in the health field, regardless of whether their concern is with "people" or "policy", do so from a strong feeling of wanting to improve things generally, for people and for society. Indeed, as philosopher David Seedhouse points out (Seedhouse, 1988), health and health promotion can probably be best seen primarily as values enterprises, with the people working in these areas believing that what they are trying to do is "good" and valuable.

These remarks bring us to consider: What *is* health promotion? What is it trying to do? There isn't an especially easy answer to these questions. But here is a first pass at it, from a "people-centred" perspective.

What is Health Promotion? What is it Trying to Do?

The most obvious response to the question "What is health promotion?" is that it is concerned with promoting health. But, in fact, this tells us very little, because almost any undertaking in the health field can fulfil this definition, even the most sickness-oriented clinical activity, which most people agree is *not* health promotion.

Historically, health promotion has referred to a domain of health activity that largely lies outside conventional treatment-oriented health service activity. As a consequence, the main players are not doctors or those directly involved in medically oriented treatment services.

Typically, discussions of health promotion make reference to health as a "positive" thing. That is, conventional treatment-oriented health services are happy to stop their interventions when symptoms have been dealt with, whereas health promoters feel there is more to one's health life than the absence of overt symptoms.

This "positive" view of health was given its initial boost by the influential definition of "health" produced by the WHO in 1948, immediately after World War II, when it was felt that the whole world was "sick". This definition says "Health is a complete state of physical, mental and social well-being, not just the absence of disease." This rather innocuous (by today's standards) definition has stirred up much controversy over the years. For example, Daniel Callahan (1990) says that the WHO definition has done more to threaten the direction and costs of health services than any other single factor. He says that, by broadening the definition beyond the absence of disease, "anything goes" in the name of health. There may be some truth to this. There are big resources in health, and a definition without clear boundaries means that it is hard to know where "health" ends and the rest of life starts.

In spite of attempts to define health positively, when one looks at most statements relating to health promotion coming out of government agencies and health authorities, the term "prevention" would probably be more accurate—that is, the concern is with reduction of disease and disabilities, rather than the promotion of health as a positive concept. And, often, there is an implicit cost-containment aspect to these statements.

Even the Lalonde Report was based on a prevention argument—that is, we have increasing rates of the diseases of affluence, which are costing our society dearly in both human and financial terms, so we have to do something about it.

In health promotion as it exists at the present time, the agendas tend to be set by policy-makers, not by those who work directly with people, and certainly not by the people themselves. And the agendas of most concern to policy-makers are undoubtedly those to do with cost containment, in particular the prevention of expensive and politically awkward diseases.

Most health promoters, in so far as they see themselves engaging in a valuable enterprise, take a different view. That is, most of us want to have positive health and well-being in society for its own sake. We want a better, happier and a more just world. We want those whose health is a problem to feel well and be well. That is why we work in the area. So the agendas of health promotion workers may be quite at variance with the agendas of "the system".

So, if we health promoters were in control, what *would* health promotion mean? What would we want to be achieving?

First, as we have said, health promotion is concerned with *positive health and well-being*. Although the prevention of disease and suffering is an aspect of this, as indeed is the relief of sickness and suffering in those who are currently sick, the whole enterprise is centred in a movement towards healthiness and wellness.

Second, and linked to what has just been said, health promotion is concerned with the *whole of life*, not just the functioning of some part of the body (such as the heart). Various terms such as "holistic", "ecological", "systems", "interdisciplinary", "intersectoral", and so on try to grasp this dimension. That is, the only realistic view to take of people and their health is one of people nested in their natural environments, particularly their everyday community settings.

Third, "health" as understood in the term "health promotion" is a *complex amalgam of bodily, mental, social and spiritual states, which on the whole change fairly slowly*. Our long-term health state tends to be established over many years, probably from childhood, and reflects the lifestyle and living-condition experiences of a lifetime. In particular, any movement towards "better health" is slow, and requires consistent input from the person or from changed environmental circumstances, or both. Therefore, the best way to view the health promotion process is as *development*—that is, as something that occurs gradually and incrementally over time.

Fourth, health promotion is concerned with *everyday life and community*. To the ordinary person, health is an experienced state, or a state observed in one's children or friends, which is an integral part of the fabric of everyday life. Getting sick, for example, has an impact on jobs, family and many other things. Being well means that one can participate in a range of activities, be energetic and worthwhile as a person, feel one can contribute without being a burden on others, and so on. Health concerns one's immediate support systems, community living, work, sex life, level of anger, ability to do the shopping, and so on. What we are really interested in here is the *long-term everyday living environment of people*—and, in a word, that adds up to *community*.

Fifth, and finally, health promotion is about a *changed balance of power in the human and health domains*. If our focus is on long-term developmental factors that determine our health status, then the question arises as to who should be directing this change process. The agendas of policy-makers and "the people" can be quite different. Which of these two should be in the driver's seat? Everyone reading this will know the answer we are looking for—the people, of course. But it is not quite as easy as that.

Certainly, we believe that the agents who should be making the key health promotion decisions, and running and owning the activities related to these decisions, should be people at the grass-roots community level, rather than the professionals and policy-makers. Much of this book is about how that can happen. Indeed, as will be seen, the "bottom line" for the kind of empowering/community development health promotion we advocate in this book is *community control*. But there are many pressures against this becoming a reality.

For one thing, many professionals find it hard to give up their power to "the community". It is pleasant to be regarded as a knowledgeable and wise helper. Here, our professional training systems have a lot to answer for, since this is what they typically set us up to expect.

And although lip-service may be paid by governmental and health agencies to concepts like participation, consultation, community boards, democracy, and so on, it is not enough for people to have theoretical control over their own health promotion destinies. Any action of value requires them to have *real decision-making power with real consequences*, and to have the *resources* to carry through the requisite action themselves. Here, we are talking in particular about money, but there are also other vital resources such as skills and knowledge, and the legislative and policy frameworks that allow self-determined action to take place. In most countries, there is very little inclination by politicians and policy-makers to give away their control, or to allow already tightly pressed health resources to go directly to "the community", which is the kind of health promotion we are talking about here. Politicians and professionals will often excuse their continuing hold on the control of things by saying that "the community" does not want to take responsibility for themselves anyway. However, our experience is generally the opposite, with "the community" typically being strongly motivated to take the kind of self-determined health promotion action this book is about. It is just that "the system" does not allow for the appropriate expression or support of this. So, on the one hand, we have "the people" wanting to take their own self-determined actions. Yet, on the other, "the system" is subtly or explicitly opposed to it.

In short, what we are talking about here is that overworked word *empowerment*. As we will discuss later, empowerment can be interpreted on a number of levels—psychological, community and societal. But behind this concept is the notion of people building their own sense of personal strength through determining their own destinies, and having the personal and material resources to do so in a supportive environment. If anything were to characterize the concept of PCHP, it would be the principle of empowerment. Although in practice there will always be a tension between the power already held by policy-makers and politicians, and the power desired by "the people", in the approach we take here we are quite clear that *the balance of power is with the people*. Health, especially those dimensions of health beyond curative medicine, is fundamentally a personal, family and community matter, and is linked closely to culture, beliefs and ways of living. Therefore it goes without saying that those with the most at stake with regard to health, and with the best capacity to make appropriate decisions and take appropriate action, are the people themselves. Obviously, people need knowledge and skills to make these decisions and to exercise their right to action. But these are simply technical matters, not insuperable barriers. Certainly, they are not reasons to justify policy-makers, professionals and academics continuing to hold most or all the power in health.

So where does all this leave us in trying to work out what health promotion is, and what it is trying to do?

In the light of what has been said here, *health promotion is an enterprise involving the development over time, in individuals and communities, of basic and positive states of and conditions for physical, mental, social and spiritual health. The control of and resources for this enterprise need to be primarily in the hands of the people themselves, but with the back-up and support of professionals, policy-makers and the overall political system.* At the heart of this enterprise are *two key concepts*: one of *development (personal and community)*, and the other of *empowerment*.

Strength-building

The term "strength-building" is one that recurs throughout this book and what we would like to do now is examine this concept.

The concept of strength-building is important not only because it is a "philosophically" sound principle, but also because it gives clear guidance as to the way in which we should work.

To make this clear, we need a little theory. Two of the disciplines informing this book are health psychology and community psychology. Both, in their own ways, deal with the concept of strength-building. Health psychology is more concerned with the individual and her or his psychology, and we will talk about this viewpoint first.

Health psychology currently uses what is called the "biopsychosocial model", which is an academic way of saying that health involves a mixture of biological, psychological and social factors. That viewpoint is nothing new, but what is interesting about this model is the picture of how these three variables are linked. Right across all health fields, increasingly it is being recognized that it is possible to talk of a general healthiness, fitness or "resistance". Some people are more susceptible to getting ill or staying well, regardless of the type of health condition concerned. All of us are more susceptible or resistant at some times than at others. For example, most people recognize that when they are run down or tired, or in a state of depression or grieving, they are more susceptible to all sorts of ailments. Likewise, when we are feeling happy or confident, we are more resistant. People who are generally optimistic have better health, and also recover better from illness (McLeod, 1986). Similarly, other research has shown that good health is related to positive psychological characteristics such as "psychological hardiness" (Kobasa et al., 1985), "self-efficacy" (Bandura, 1977), "self-esteem" (Cohen and Lazarus, 1983), a "sense of coherence" (Antonovsky, 1987), "personal control" (Steptoe and Appels, 1989), and so on. It appears that the "psychologically stronger" people feel, the better their health. What is more, it appears that this psychological strength can be developed by anyone. There are various ways of doing this, but they can probably be summed up as "personal empowerment". That is, regardless of the actual specific knowledge or skills involved, if people are engaged in activities, and live in environments, which enhance their capabilities, their confidence, their self-esteem, their sense of control, their competence, and the regard in which others hold them, then their health is likely to be enhanced.

Closely linked to the psychological strength-building idea is that of social support. For many years, both medicine and psychology functioned as though people were islands—that is, as bodies or minds that have minimal or no contact with other people. The fact of the matter is that people are, above all else, social beings. Even those who are very private or isolated are "social", in the sense that the "social deprivation" they impose on themselves or find themselves in often appears to have quite a major health cost. It is clear that people's sense of control or personal empowerment is closely linked to their support systems (Cohen and Syme, 1985). To the extent that people feel supported emotionally and practically, they also tend to feel strong. Also, the development of the requisite knowledge and skills that lead to the individual's developing his or her strengths is almost always best done in group settings. People typically learn better and more happily with others than, say, alone with a home study course, although the latter can work too. Overall, then, the concept of strength-building is inseparable from the concept of social support and social context, even though the principal "academic" focus in psychology and medicine still tends to remain on the individual largely divorced from his or her living context. In particular, as we will see, the concept of *participation* is especially relevant for health promotion of the kind we advocate here.

With regard to the "biological" component of the biopsychosocial complex, there are some interesting aspects relevant to our discussion here too. For example, there is increasing interest in the field called psychoneuroimmunology, which concerns the relationship between psychological factors and the immune system (Locke et al., 1985). Research into the immune system is happening at a high rate around the world, although the investigation of the role of psychological factors is still in its relative infancy. Nevertheless, it is clear that the status of the immune system, which pervades the whole body, and operates at the molecular level, is vital for general health, and has an important role in determining susceptibility to cancer, infections and other diseases. In general, the functioning of the immune system is responsive to both positive and negative psychological changes, with factors such as stress being especially important.

Likewise, in the area of cardiovascular health, it has long been recognized that there are important links with psychological variables. In general, cardiovascular health is at least in part determined by factors such as stress, coping style (as in Type A behaviour), a sense of control, and so on (Sarafino, 1994). Social support has also been found to be an important variable in heart health (Lynch, 1977).

What we have just been talking about shows that there are interesting linkages between psychological, social and biological factors in a way that is relevant to health promotion concerns. In general, it can be concluded that if people are feeling strong, and are in a supportive and stable environment, then their physical health is likely to be enhanced. There is similar evidence for mental and social health. On a wide variety of measures, mental health is found to be better when people feel efficacious, strong and socially supported (Pransky, 1991). Likewise, social health indicators such as violence, abuse, suicide, family breakdown, and so on are closely linked to similar factors.

As for community psychology, it has long been quite explicit that "strength-building" means much the same thing as "empowerment" (Rappaport, 1987). Typically, in community psychology, the focus is on building social support and building community. The research evidence is that the better the community one lives in from a "socially supportive" and "cohesion" point of view, the better the health of the people in it.

To sum up, then, the concept of strength-building is used here to show us how to work in a health-promoting way. To the extent that our activities build strengths (skills, knowledge, competencies, self-esteem, power, social support, etc.), then they can be regarded as health-promoting. To the extent that they detract from people's strength (where others have control over our lives, where there are poor living conditions and inadequate resources, where people are put down, where there is high unemployment, where cultural or community disruption takes place, where opportunities are lacking, where social support is absent, etc.), then poor health will almost inevitably be the result. Indeed, there is some evidence that this may be the single most important factor in determining overall health status of people (Syme, 1989).

HOW DOES THIS APPLY TO YOU?

It is assumed that the readers of this book are either currently "doers" of health promotion (either as professionals or community people), or wanting to be doers (that is, students). So how does what we have been saying apply to you?

As stated before, we feel that the majority of our existing training systems generally do not equip students and professionals to work in a strength-building and empowering way. The assumption is, in most educational approaches, that the trained person will know best, and we (the experts) will "do to" the client or community. Clearly, this is an inappropriate approach if one is to practise PCHP.

Because health promotion now covers so many disciplines and professions, it is hard to make assumptions about the backgrounds of students of health promotion. And because differing backgrounds will probably mean that people will work in different settings, then it is hard to be too specific about examples. In spite of this, we believe there is a general approach that can be used here, which is embodied in terms such as "strength-building", "empowerment", "community development" and "personal development". This approach is applicable by almost any kind of health promotion worker in almost any setting, and in any group of people with whom one is working, whether that be a family, a small group, or a whole community, and whether those people are currently "sick" or "well". We also believe these principles can be applied in whole populations and countries, and hope that one day they will be (see Chapter 15).

To sum up, then, the broad principles underlying our people-centred approach to health promotion can be stated as follows:

1. Health promotion is concerned first and foremost with real, living people, not abstract policies or statistics.
2. It is distinct from most prevailing health and medical practice by emphasizing positive, life-enhancing matters, not just the removal of negativities such as symptoms or social problems.
3. The perspective is inevitably one of gradual change over time, best characterized by the word "development". Here, the terms "community development" and "personal development" are the closest to what we want.
4. The best methods to use are those that can be regarded as "strength-building"—that is, they are aimed at developing people's strengths, skills, knowledge and resources. The focus is on strengths, not weaknesses or problems.
5. It is important to be systematic and well organized in these endeavours, and to be clear about needs, wishes, goals, resources, management and evaluation processes.
6. Behind everything we do are important philosophical values, best characterized by terms such as "empowerment", "justice", "equity", "cultural appropriateness" and "spirituality". Ultimately, what we are after is a better life for as many people as possible on their own terms, and in particular a better life for those who currently tend to miss out.
7. Finally, it is also important to be clear that our concern is with "health", as distinct from other worthwhile social and justice endeavours. Ultimately, our work is oriented to those outcomes which can readily be accepted as having primarily a health dimension, in particular physical health and mental health.

As we proceed in this book, we will return to all these matters, and we hope that, by the time you have finished, you will feel 'empowered' to go out and engage in a people-centred, strength-building form of health promotion that will be satisfying to you, and of benefit to those with whom you work.

2

PEOPLE-CENTRED HEALTH PROMOTION
The Key Essentials

In Chapter 1, we covered broad issues relating to health promotion generally, and to a more "people-centred" approach to health promotion. In this chapter, we want to outline what we are calling "People-Centred Health Promotion" (PCHP). To do this, we use the mnemonic "PEOPLE" as a convenient starting point. (In a sense, this chapter summarizes everything the book is about.)

> People-centredness
> Empowerment
> Organizational and community development
> Participation
> Life quality
> Evaluation

P: PEOPLE-CENTREDNESS

It goes without saying that a PCHP is people-centred. But what does this mean? We see such a health promotion approach as beginning with the everyday experience of people, from the perspective of their natural community settings. As far as professionals are concerned, their role needs to be one which honours this perspective. We now look at this in more detail.

Everyday Experience

In so far as health promotion is an academic or "scientific" exercise, then it is possible to contrast health promotion as a field with other social science and health endeavours. For most of these, the standard approach is some variation of what is called "positivism", where the subjects of research are viewed as objects to be studied by a dispassionate observer or measuring instrument, and where the data are collected from an external and non-subjective viewpoint. For example, in psychology, subjective or experiential data have until recently typically been regarded as suspect and, in most health sciences, "statistics" or data based on clearly identifiable, unarguable events or objects (which can readily be counted) have always been the preference.

Hence, to argue that a respectable field of social science or health science be based primarily in experiential data or subjectivity is to be on somewhat precarious ground. Yet there is a growing movement in social science that supports this way of going about things. The sort of research stance involved here is described by terms such as "qualitative", "constructivist", "post-modernist" or "phenomenological", all ways of saying that it is possible to get good information by asking people about how they see the world, and how they feel about things. Obviously, this kind of research approach would have much to offer health promotion, and this viewpoint has been strongly advocated now for several years (e.g. Maclean and Eakin, 1992).

We are not arguing that *all* research or information-gathering should be of this nature. What we are saying is that the starting point of health promotion as a formal endeavour should be the world view, the way of experiencing the world, of actual people—not the inferences drawn from "objective data" gathered by dispassionate outsiders.

Also, in most health science research, the representation of people is typically dehumanized. Even when people rather than statistics are mentioned, terms such as "subjects", "interviewees", "patients", "clients", etc. tend to distance the reader from what is going on, and to make the people involved seem like disembodied, lifeless objects divorced from their everyday surroundings. We feel that the whole language and way of looking at people in health promotion need to reflect the fact that we are all real human beings of value, and capable of thought, feelings, intelligent action and even nobility!

Of all the social sciences, psychology is the one which is closest to dealing with people's actual experience, reflected in terms such as "consciousness", "cognition", "emotions", "appraisal", "perception", and so on. From that point of view, we will draw strongly on psychology as an academic base for PCHP, although other disciplines such as sociology and anthropology make important contributions as well.

The point we are making here about starting with people's experience as the basis for our study was made eloquently by E. E. Sampson in an article entitled "The democratization of psychology" (Sampson, 1991), which argues for an experiential base for psychology. In that article, Sampson cites research by Lave (1988), who coined the term jpf's, or "just plain folks", to represent ordinary human beings in psychological research. Lave was interested in the psychology of arithmetical computation, and looked at people doing simple addition tasks under laboratory conditions compared with adding up prices or calculating amounts in a supermarket. What she found was that, although the arithmetical task was similar in both settings, the strategies used by people in each setting were quite different. That is, jpf's in their everyday settings operate differently from those same folks in a laboratory setting. Since most of psychology is based on laboratory research, it is possible that a substantial proportion of the conclusions drawn by academic psychologists for the past 100 years have been erroneous, or at least off track, in terms of how people operate in everyday life. One cannot draw too sweeping conclusions from Lave's work, but it stands as a nice metaphor.

Community Perspective

Not only do we need to start with the experience of people, but also that experience needs to be grounded in the ordinary, everyday contexts in which we all find ourselves. In health promotion, one is not dealing with people in a clinic or laboratory, but in real life, in the community. The way we operate in our everyday lives, what we do from day to day, how we think and feel, interact with others, deal with stress, and so on all profoundly affect our health. This is the context of health promotion—the daily round, the household, the workplace, the neighbourhood, our networks—and so any study or practice involving health promotion should reflect this.

The concept of "community" recurs frequently through this book and, to the despair of many academics, it is a term that can take on many meanings. We make no apology for using the term in a variety of ways. However, we will attempt to define what we mean by it in these different usages. Here, a "community perspective" is different from the perspective adopted by most health and social science. That is, the usual "scientific" approach is either to study people divorced from their settings, or to have those settings described in the most minimal of terms. Here, "community" means "everyday setting", the nexus in which people live out their lives from moment to moment, and which, for most of us, involves the rather mundane issues of the house we live in, family, relationships, neighbourhood, workplace, school, church, interest groups, clubs, community services, local politics, and so on. Social scientists often like to be "lordly" and remote. Here we are attempting to reverse that trend, and bring the discourse down to the intimate and ordinary details of everyday life and situation, including people's psychological reactions to, and interactions with, these situations. This is why the previous point about experience—people's subjectivity—is so important, because it is the *perception* of situations rather than their objective reality that research repeatedly shows is crucial for health-related issues.

Facilitatory Role for Professionals

The whole stance of positivism and a remote, non-people perspective that has characterized much social science reinforces a view that the social scientist is a supreme being, who observes god-like the doings of a depersonalized and abstract common mob. As many writers have pointed out, professionals generally form an élite, who feel their language, way of looking at things and analysis are somehow superior to those of ordinary people. On the whole, professionals simply do not trust ordinary people, seeing them as lacking knowledge, living inappropriate lifestyles, absconding with resources, and generally not doing what they should to keep themselves healthy. The more social-structural of social scientists often tend to discount the power of individuals and people-as-people, often implying they are mere puppets in the face of implacable (and usually negative) social forces that constantly threaten their health and well-being, whether these be oppression, poor housing, capitalism, communism, a polluted environment, bad policy, or anything else. In short, the professional analysis tends to be that the viewpoint of ordinary people is of little account.

In PCHP, we take the opposite stance. We argue that the greatest wisdom is held by ordinary people, that professionals often only serve to mess people up when they interfere with natural processes, and that, certainly, professional arrogance about the superiority of their views is totally unjustified. Not only is the traditional professional view an incorrect one (i.e. that they have superior knowledge), but it is also very disempowering. As will be seen shortly, empowerment is *the* basic value in PCHP, and this means power that is developed and experienced and held by jpf's. Not only does a facilitatory role for professionals mean that we acknowledge that the jpf's are in charge, but it also means backing up and supporting what it is they (the jpf's) decide to do. This may mean finding appropriate resources, bringing knowledge and skills into the community, being available when requested, and generally being a positive and helpful presence. This is a very rewarding role once one gets into it.

However, most professional training does not support this approach. Rather, it tends to reinforce the view that professionals are a special race, to whom due deference should be given by the unwashed masses. A principal aim of this book is to provide a resource that puts another view, and which can be used in training and learning situations to start creating a different kind of professional. Indeed, many professionals *do* work in the kind of way we are talking about here, but sadly not enough. Also, the professional-superiority ethos permeates the system so universally that even the best-intentioned professional is subtly or not so subtly affected by it. We are only human, and it is natural to want the power and prestige that goes with professionalism.

Notwithstanding that, what we are hoping to do here is provide a basis for a new kind of professionalism, one where professionals work as facilitators. What does working as a facilitator mean? It means making the mental shift to acknowledging that the people we are working with are in charge, and that we are there to offer our skills and ideas to the extent that those people want to use them, and generally to help in the process of making things happen, as those people want them to happen. This does not mean, as some think, that as professionals we have to be backward or passive in our role—we can be as upfront and noisy as we want. But it is within a framework that assumes that the people we are working with are in control. And, here, it is worth emphasizing that by "people" we mean, whenever possible, ordinary grass-roots people, not just some professional further down the pecking order. It may not always be possible to achieve this, but this is the aim.

This is not the place to elaborate further on these matters, and we will come back repeatedly throughout this book to how this facilitatory principle operates in practice. Indeed, it is a lot of what the book is about. But it is probably important at this point to address a couple of the most frequently voiced objections to this approach. One of these is that people do not have the knowledge required to make appropriate decisions, and to run their own activities. The answer to this is that PCHP is, by its nature, a developmental enterprise, requiring extended periods of time, and that part of this enterprise is ensuring that the knowledge base is there for people to make good decisions, and to undertake optimal action. The experience we have had working in this way has shown us that this approach works, and the long-term results are typically superior to, and more enduring than, what is typically accomplished by professionals who work in the old, top-down way. However, the price to be paid for these results in any major project is for the people involved to go through a preliminary phase of building knowledge and an appropriate values base.

One other explicit or implicit criticism by professionals of the kind of approach we are advocating is that people are not to be trusted. One variation of this is that, if resources are brought into a community, pressure groups, "the middle class", or unscrupulous people will co-opt those resources, so that we end up with a project that is under the control of a minority, or with the resources having been squandered. Admittedly there are dangers here. However, provided there are very clear constitutional guidelines about what is being done, and a constant awareness of these dangers, our experience is that they do not happen. Or if they do start to happen, they can be corrected. The bottom line of this approach is *trust*, and our experience is that most people can be trusted, although there will be exceptions as in any field of endeavour. Indeed, it can be asserted with some confidence that professionals are not necessarily any more trustworthy than jpf's. Also, there can be just as many checks and balances in a community environment as in a supposedly "ethical" professional organization.

Summary

To sum up, then, "people-centredness" means that our health promotion enterprise is driven by a viewpoint that starts with the actual subjective experience of ordinary people, rather than with the "objective" views of social scientists looking at abstract data. In particular, the subjective experience of most interest is that of people in their everyday community settings. As professionals working in terms of these imperatives, we need to change from the traditional "top-down" way of looking at things to an approach we characterize as "facilitatory".

E: EMPOWERMENT

Empowerment is the basic philosophical tenet of this whole approach. In Chapter 5, we will explore the concept of empowerment in more detail. Here, we will just sketch out broadly what we mean by this term.

The term "empowerment" has been a catchword in health promotion now for many years. Notwithstanding that, it is rare to find it fully operational as a principle. PCHP as presented here attempts to carry this principle to its ultimate practical limit and, in so doing, takes it out of the realm of rhetoric into its real-life manifestation.

So what do we mean by "empowerment"? Here, it is seen first and foremost as having to do with control. This control relates both to whatever endeavour is being undertaken, and to the psychological strength and sense of mastery people get from the processes and the fruits of the enterprise. It also involves what we characterize as a "strength-building approach" and a "resource-based approach". We now look at these areas in more detail.

Control

The cornerstone of empowerment is the concept of control. We break control down into three main categories:

1. Community Control

Here, the term "community" refers to sectors of population represented by ordinary people, by jpf's, as distinct from official, political, professional, bureaucratic or institutional power structures. Communities may be geographically based, or they may be interest based. What counts in this definition is that they are groupings of people who do not have a lot of ready-made power in terms of existing organizational strength. (Here the role of existing community or voluntary organizations may need special attention as to whether they qualify.) The primary *raison d'être* of such groupings is the strength that the people in them actually or potentially get from other people with whom they are in immediate contact through virtue of their membership in the same community. In short, it is the people-network aspect of the grouping that is the central defining issue, together with its "people feel". To the extent that a health promotion "project" is involving a definable grouping in the community, and this community fits the general picture given here, then it is desirable that that grouping be as broad based and as representative as possible. In short, "generic" community rather than focused special interest groups are of most interest. (However, most communities are made up of subgroupings, and we turn to these in a moment.)

Since, by definition, the kind of community alluded to is that which does not currently have a lot of "power" when compared with other power blocs in society, it is very easy for professionals and officialdom to feel that they have "power over" that community. So the central point here is that, right from the beginning, a firm commitment is made to the principle that, whatever happens, the final control is in the hands of the people of interest—the community to be affected by the health promotion undertaking. How this is accomplished will become clearer as the book proceeds. However, here it is sufficient to say that such community control requires four main steps. The first is that, *constitutionally* (that is, in an agreed-on, written-down form), a commitment is made to community control, and the structures are described to ensure that this happens. The second is that, *organizationally*, attention is given to how the enterprise will be run in practice, so that the control is unambiguously in the hands of the community concerned. The third is that, *developmentally*, the project is evolved carefully with checks and balances in place to ensure the maintenance of community control. In addition, to the extent that professionals are involved, they will need to know how to work this way, and it may also be necessary to have internal training programmes to help community people develop the necessary skills to fulfil the roles and functions required by this approach. Finally, *evaluation systems* need to be in place to ensure that community control, typically a fragile affair until fully established on an enduring basis, is actually happening and continues to happen.

2. Group Control

As mentioned above, most communities are composed of subgroups, some of which are "natural" (such as families, neighbourhoods, villages and tribes), some "manufactured" but pre-existing (such as societies, workplaces, clubs, associations, voluntary agencies, churches, and established self-help groups), and some "manufactured" as the result of health promotion initiatives in which one might be involved. To the extent that any of these groups are seen as fundamental to a health promotion project, then people will relate to that group strongly within the framework of the project.

Each group is likely to have its own life, goals, network, loyalties, and so on, and therefore becomes a vital part of any health promotion enterprise. To the extent that the group feels autonomous, effective, in charge of its own affairs, and able to set its own agenda, then it will be "empowered". The aim, then, is to be aware of these groupings, and to ensure that, as far as possible, they are enabled to make their own decisions and run their own affairs. Obviously, there may be interchange with a larger "community" and with professionals and other officials. But the aim should always be for that group to decide its own destiny as far as possible, with resources and back-up available to it as required.

3. Personal Control

As mentioned in Chapter 1, health psychology is currently interested in a psychological variable called "personal control", which is seen as a central factor in determining health and illness status. This variable takes on a variety of names, such as self-efficacy, a sense of coherence, competence, personal effectiveness, good coping skills, and so on. Basically, it refers to how well people feel they cope in different, especially difficult, situations, and the general sense of mastery that results from this. The variable seems to rely on at least two factors: one is a sense of autonomy or independence—that the person can rely on her or himself rather than depend on others to get them through situations. The other is the level of skill or knowledge that person has in relation to a situation—that is, the "strength" they have to cope with a situation.

We return to consider personal control further in Chapter 5. Here, we just want to say that this is an important dimension for the present discussion, since it seems to be a broad personal attribute that has a direct link to the health of the body and mind, and which also has a direct link to the more global sorts of empowerment we have just been discussing. In short, an empowering environment is likely to lead to a sense of personal control, which in turn is likely to be beneficial to health.

Strength-building Approach

In Chapter 1, we mentioned community psychologist Julian Rappaport's writing on the topic of empowerment in terms of strength-building (Rappaport, 1987). Rappaport contrasts strength-building with the traditional deficit-oriented approaches typically used in psychology and other health sciences and clinical practices. That is, most orthodox practices approach human problems by assessing and attempting to treat deficits (symptoms, illness, specific problems, risk factors, etc.). A strength-building approach, however, is oriented to assets. By building on assets or strengths—a positive approach—the negativities or deficits are seen to take care of themselves. The two approaches lead to quite different strategies and outcomes. For example, people who experience strength-building generally acquire new and lasting skills and knowledge, which can be applied in future situations—quite different from most who simply get "treated" for a problem. Also, the aim of a strength-building approach is increased self-esteem and personal control, and these changes in turn often "empower" people to tackle other life areas, and to go on improving the overall situation for themselves and others.

It can be seen that personal control and strength-building are closely linked concepts. However, whereas personal control is an "outcome", strength-building is more descriptive of a process. This is an important point, because *strength-building* is the underlying process for almost every aspect of PCHP.

Strength-building is not just a concept that applies at the personal level. It also applies at the group and whole community level. At the group level, it means finding out who can do what in a group, then building on these resources to develop a strong group ethos and a sense of well-being and power in that group. At the community level, strength-building also means searching for the assets, resources and key effective people in a community, and building on those. Any community, no matter how downtrodden or demoralized, has talented people with skills. This approach means finding those people and using them for the benefit of the whole community. The result is that the growth comes from within the community, and is hence under their control, rather than from some remote outside source, which can also create dependencies, the opposite of autonomy and control.

Overall, then, strength-building signifies a general way of working that we see as being at the heart of PCHP. Rather than looking for target problems and target groups to rectify, which is a typical approach of much health promotion, we look for assets and strengths that can be developed and maintained. This leads, in turn, to the consideration of a *resource-based approach* to health promotion.

Resource-based Approach

The conventional way for professionals to work with people is for those professionals to be seen as the repository of special skills and knowledge, and for the people to be the fortunate recipients of those skills and that knowledge. With this approach, the power clearly remains with the professional. In PCHP, with its emphasis on empowerment, professional knowledge and skills are there to be shared with the community. To the extent that the community can have access to these resources, it is empowered to take its own action and to be master or mistress of its own destiny. The enemy of empowerment is *dependency*—where people come to depend on others, often experts, for what they can or cannot do. Our aim is to develop a climate that is the opposite of dependency, where people feel strong, independent, in control, self-determining, and so on.

At the basis of this as a strategic approach is the concept of accessible resources that are available in a form, language and cost structure for easy use by a community. Resources enable people to remain in control of their activities, and to be free to do what they want (including rejecting those resources if they wish). Very often, some expert back-up will be required for resources to be utilized properly, or at least will be required in the initial stages of developing or using a resource. But this is quite different from the professional being the repository of "specialist" and "secret" knowledge that only he or she possesses. As said before, we favour the professional as "facilitator" rather than as "little god".

The term "resources" may mean knowledge and skills, as we have been using it here, or it may, of course, mean money and facilities, or access to decision-making. As far as professionals are concerned, the same principles apply. That is, often professionals will have access to financial resources such as grants, and access to political and other power structures in a way that is difficult or impossible for ordinary community people to have. The professional who works in a resource-based, strength-building way will assist the community to get access to those resources by helping it to do its own applications and advocate for itself, rather than disempower people by doing those things for them. Constantly, many of us who are professionals have to fight against our natural "helping" instincts, and we have to be careful that our well-intentioned "helping" is not doing people a long-term disservice.

Summary

The concept of empowerment is seen as the fundamental philosophical principle of PCHP. It is defined here in practical terms as involving control over life affairs, at the community, group and personal level. This control is established by a process of strength-building at these various levels, accomplished through people having access to the knowledge, skill, material and political resources needed to give them control over, and the ability to undertake, the decisions and activities they deem to be appropriate in a health promotion context.

O: ORGANIZATIONAL AND COMMUNITY DEVELOPMENT

PCHP involves *people* rather than individuals—that is, people in their collectivity, rather than as isolated persons. Therefore, the whole basis of the approach is grounded in people doing things together. Not only is this realistic in terms of the way most of us, as social animals, conduct our daily lives, but also it enables the health promoter to capitalize on the powerful processes, supports and benefits of group and community work.

Of recent years, the term "community development" has become almost as much a catchphrase in health promotion as "empowerment". But like empowerment, the term means different things to different people. Here, we are quite clear about what it means. That is, the community development we are talking about is based broadly on principles of organizational development. In what follows in this section, we go over briefly what this means. In Chapter 6, we go into these issues in more detail.

Organizational Development

The approach to community development to be outlined here is not exclusively from the area known as organizational development (OD), but the model outlined in OD is as clear an exposition as one can get. Also, the OD approach can be applied to any aggregation of people, community or otherwise, so is a good general model to know about.

OD is typically used in industry and other such settings, where performance, productivity and morale are issues, and one wants to have an optimally functioning organization, with a high level of cohesion, well-being and satisfaction on the part of all those involved. As may be seen, this model can well apply to a community, where the aim is the attainment of certain objectives in the best kind of way, and in whose members there is also a desire to develop cohesiveness and well-being.

According to Van de Ven and Poole (1995), OD is a change process, or "a progression of change events that unfold during the duration of an entity's existence". Increasingly, this is a perspective that finds acceptance in the OD literature and in health promotion efforts in organizations.

Moreover, the view about what is most likely to produce "healthy change" in organizations seems to be shifting toward a people-centred approach. For example, the "new paradigm of work", which has evolved over the past few decades, has involved a shift from authoritarian and hierarchical corporate structures to "community corporate" and "team-building" models (Maynard and Merhten, 1995). This has meant that many organizations have moved toward structures emphasizing employee empowerment and continual learning at all levels.

This approach has been characterized by Peter Senge as "the learning organization" (Senge, 1994). According to him, "the organizations that will excel in years to come will be those that understand how to gain the commitment of employees at all levels and continually expand their capacity to learn". Such an approach is certainly consistent with the principles of PCHP and has implications for community development.

In particular, Senge suggests that there are five disciplines practised by "learning organizations": systems thinking; personal mastery; mental models; shared vision; and team learning. "Systems thinking" is a conceptual framework that encourages people within an organization to see patterns of organizational behaviour, and learn to reinforce or change them effectively. "Personal mastery" has to do with working energetically towards a vision that is based on an understanding of organizational behaviour. "Mental models" are defined as the way in which "we understand the world and take action in it based on notions that reside deeply in the psyche". "Shared vision" has to do with goals, values and missions shared throughout the organization, which include, but go beyond, the written vision statement. Finally, "team learning" means a commitment of the organization to working together in such a way that the learning of the whole team is greater than that of the individual members (Senge, 1994).

Others working in the OD field have suggested that what is most conducive to supporting the empowerment of employees are environments that are seen by employees as having a participatory culture and a consistent vision and message to them affirming their importance to the success of the organization (Spreitzer, 1995). Senior managers who are participatory in their management style are seen as essential to creating such a culture. Such approaches have been found to have beneficial effects for the organization and the individuals involved. For example, studies have found employees who have a sense of ownership and responsibility to be more motivated, productive and healthier (e.g. Howlett and Archer, 1984; Weissman, 1982).

The principles and approaches of OD are not new to the health promotion field. For example, Canada has developed an approach to health promotion in the workplace called the Workplace Health System (WHS), which incorporates many of these principles and approaches. Specifically, the WHS attempts to achieve a value consensus from the people involved in the organization (including the workers), tries to find out what these people want, and attempts to develop a plan jointly agreed upon by management and workers which is matched to resources. This system also uses evaluation and feedback as a means of understanding the process and adapting it to changes in the environment.

Overall, then, we feel that OD is a field with a great deal to contribute to PCHP, in particular as this relates to community development.

Community Development

In Chapter 6, the topic of community development is discussed at length. Here, we want to say that we see community development as involving (broadly) the application of OD principles to a whole community (locality or interest, though we favour locality), in the context of a philosophy of empowerment and of objectives relating to health-related quality of life (see below). The process is geared to mobilizing whole communities to work together on goals, to build strengths and to foster community cohesiveness and spirit, all within an evaluative and self-correcting framework. More specifically, the following are seen to be essential steps in a PCHP community development process:

1. Participatory formulation of a philosophy of action for the enterprise and of the overall objectives.
2. Participatory planning for action through seeking representative information from the community of concern about their needs, wishes and views on potential strategies.
3. Consensual setting of clearly stated, prioritized, time-limited goals, which attempt to combine the essentials of what is derived from the information-gathering process with the overall philosophy of the enterprise. These goals are in a form that directs action, guides resource decisions, and provides a basis for the evaluation of process and outcome.
4. Consensually agreed-on resource plans and resource allocation, in terms of the established priorities and goals.
5. Allocation of tasks to clearly specified people willing to do them, and action involving as many participants as possible, with the aim of both meeting goals and forming social bonds.
6. Regular review of all major project goals and processes in a public forum, to correct goals and strategies where necessary and to reinforce and support successful action.
7. Periodic assessment of outcomes, using a variety of indices, to determine the overall status of the project and its effectiveness from a goal-attainment, health and community point of view, with the aim of

providing data for accountability, getting further resources, and for generally summing up and confirming the directions taken.

In addition to the above, the overall management of the community enterprise is seen as one which is empowering, "bottom up", and driven by community needs, wishes and values. The issue of management and the community development procedural steps outlined briefly here are addressed in detail in Part III, together with examples of their application.

P: PARTICIPATION

The terms "participation" and "participants" were used several times above, and they represent what is generally thought to be a "good thing" in health promotion. For example, the 1986 Canadian government document *Achieving health for all: A framework for health promotion* (Epp, 1986) puts a high value on what it calls "public participation". However, we have to be sure that we are clear what "participation" really means, and why it *is* a good thing, if it is not to become just another meaningless political word. For example, in some contexts, it can simply mean token top-down consultation with an unrepresentative group from a "community", the input of whom may then be ignored anyway.

So, in terms of PCHP, what is participation, and is it a "good thing"? The answer to the second question is an emphatic "Yes", provided certain conditions are fulfilled.

1. Involvement of as Many People as Possible

In a PCHP context, the central focus is, of course, people. On the whole, the view we take in PCHP of "people" is in their aggregation as a "community". Such a community has at least two characteristics. One is that the larger the community, the more diverse it is likely to be. For example, most modern geographic communities, unless they are specifically catering for a certain sector of the population such as the retired, will have in them a wide diversity of people, with this diversity related to factors such as ethnicity, gender, age, income, education, religion, social class, sexual preference, or whatever. The other characteristic of most communities, especially larger ones, is that although people will be diverse, this diversity is likely to be organized into groups where like attracts like. And smaller groups (such as a family) will tend to join larger groups (such as a neighbourhood) because of factors shared in common with others.

PCHP honours diversity. In common with community psychology, it explicitly adopts diversity as a positive value to be pursued, not only because this accepts the reality of most community situations and does not try to impose a single set of values on to a given situation, but also because it is seen as lending strength to the overall society. One dimension of diversity that we feel needs special emphasis in PCHP is culture, and Chapter 7 is devoted to that topic. Our strength as a society is seen as coming not from homogeneity, but from diversity. Of course, if that diversity is so pronounced that people are fighting amongst themselves, then the society is weakened. A "transcendent goal" of PCHP is the paradoxical one of a unity based both on our shared humanity and community, and on a respecting of differences between people that means we do not try to change each other. Accepting people as they are recognizes their existing strengths and assets, rather than regarding their "difference" as a "problem". However, it is acknowledged that almost all the serious problems of societies, be they war, class tension, racial conflict, religious bigotry, prejudice, violence, or other such matters, typically have in them an element of one group's not accepting the values and habits of another group, and hence trying to change or overwhelm them. What we are talking about here is a very important and complex social phenomenon, and is at the heart of a "true" sense of community, and also of the kind of peaceful, constructive and enjoyable society most people want.

The recognition of diversity, however, means that a goal of participation becomes quite difficult. That is, the conventional "prevention" method of singling out a target group and focusing on a specific problem or related set of problems is by definition a non-honouring of diversity. It is deliberately seeking a homogeneous situation. That is not what we want to pursue here. Rather, we believe that we are seeking a balance between recognizing the important differences between people, while attempting to transcend these in a common cause of "community". The fact of the matter is that we do have to live together, so we might as well live together as well as we can.

"Participation" in a PCHP sense, then, becomes a matter of trying to engage as many groups and sectors of an overall community as possible. This means using labels in a light-touch way—enough to recognize a "distinct grouping", but not so much that it encourages a hard and fast boundary. Such boundaries typically lead to an "out-group" attitude on the part of members of other groupings, which, as was shown in early social psychology experiments (e.g. Sherif, 1966), often then leads to negative labelling and hostility. (Terms like "teenagers", "smokers", "environmentalists" or names of ethnic groups can easily go this way.)

In short, from a community perspective (where "community" is seen as an aggregation of groupings of people linked by common geography and/or interest, and capable of seeing each other as part of a common "whole"), it is desirable to have as many people as possible in that community engaged in a health promotion endeavour. The aim is maximal participation, and to have the undertaking erring on the side of inclusiveness rather than exclusiveness. All groups in a community have something to offer, and all groups can learn from others. It is this philosophy that underlies our participation perspective.

2. Representativeness

Not only does one want participation in terms of numbers and variety, one also wants *representativeness*. That is, it is often said that those who benefit most from health promotion activities are those that need them least. Those "most in need" are generally also those who are the most disempowered in terms of education, financial resources, political power, self-esteem, and so on, and who may tend not to come forward if things are left on a purely voluntary basis. The traditional answer to this is, once again, target groups. That is, if some group or groups are identified as being the most problematical, and are labelled as such, then efforts are "targeted" at them to make them change their errant ways, or to otherwise rectify their problem. As we hope may now be seen, this is not consonant with the philosophy we are espousing here. Rather, the alternative and more positive approach is to assume that everyone in a community will be involved, each bringing his or her strengths to the issues at hand. On this assumption, as will be seen shortly, the key to getting participation in a PCHP community development framework is needs assessment/information-gathering that really taps into people's motivation, and which captures the essence of what they want for themselves, so that they will be irresistibly drawn into getting involved. The key to representativeness, then, is needs assessment/information-gathering that goes out of its way to include the views of those who are otherwise not heard. It may require a combination of sampling, ethnographic, interviewing and community organizational efforts to ensure that this goal of representative information-gathering is achieved. Certainly, since it is a difficult area, it needs to remain high in the consciousness of those organizing health promotion endeavours, so that the goal of a voice for everyone is achieved.

Once it has been found what people at all levels of the community want for themselves, the next step is the art of setting appropriate goals for activities that will encourage the participation of all sectors of the community (and at this stage, some low-key "targeting" may be required, so that one ensures that certain groups are catered for). Then the activities themselves need to be advertised and presented in such a way (including such factors as location and cost) that the potential participation of those normally shy about coming forward is optimized.

3. Popular Activities that Motivate, Meet Needs and Strengthen

This factor has already been alluded to in the context of ensuring participation by all sectors of a community. However, the point needs to be made separately that the ultimate factor in a successful, participatory community health promotion project is the design and implementation of activities that are attractive to the members of that community. To meet this criterion, they need to be attuned to the expressed needs and wishes of the community, and to be in accord with the recommended strategies for meeting needs obtained in the information-gathering process. As well, the activities themselves need to be of high quality, well organized, clear in their goals, friendly, fun (if possible), socially supportive, and generally rewarding for the participants. An important aim in any community activity is that not only are people doing something they feel is worthwhile, but also they are strengthening the social bonds between them through their involvement. Indeed, we believe that all PCHP community-based activities need to have this double agenda—of worthwhile activity and social-bond building.

It also goes without saying that all activities need to be empowering, which has a lot to do with both leadership and process. In particular, it is important that activity leaders work in a facilitatory rather than an autocratic way. An important aspect of the empowerment agenda in activities is that people emerge from each participatory episode, and from the whole experience, feeling strengthened. This may mean having acquired new knowledge or skills, having made new friends, feeling more in control, having a higher level of well-being and self-esteem, and so on. In short, the aim is a higher quality of life, which we address in the next section.

At this stage, readers may be asking: What is actually meant by "activities"? Give us some examples! In one way, it is a pity to do this, because there is virtually a limitless number of types of PCHP activities. However, a random list of examples could be such things as: working together on building community facilities; setting up preschool activities; holiday programmes for children; craft classes; personal development activities such as stress management and communication skill building; lifestyle change activities such as weight control; planning and developing cooperative community work programmes; enhancing cultural awareness in a community; workshops on parenting skills; a cooperative gardening programme; learning one's legal rights; a village on a South Pacific island planning a healthy eating campaign; economic development in a Third World rural community; increasing school children's awareness of the need for exercise; building safe neighbourhoods; budgeting skills; self-help groups to do with women's issues; anger management; learning a new language; and so on, and so on. The important thing is that, in a health promotion context, such activities are seen as having direct relevance to health and well-being, and that the outcomes of participation in these activities are assessed in these terms (among other things).

Why, you might ask, would learning a new language have an impact on health? Or learning budgeting skills? Here we make the proposition that participation in strength-building, socially supportive, empowering activities of almost any nature is good for one's health and well-being. One feels more in control, which as we noted before, has been shown to be beneficial to one's health. One also feels oneself to be an integral part of a community (shown by various authors to be good for cardiovascular and other health). Group activities of the type described here engender social support, for which a substantial research literature shows positive health and mental health benefits. Generally, activities that start to get people to look at their own lives, and to mobilize their energies in a new and developmental direction, are likely to whet an interest in self-improvement and life enhancement, which in turn is likely to have a health dimension. As many studies have found, once people start to change one aspect of their lives, they begin to improve and take action in other areas as well, either deliberately or as a side-benefit. Ideally, of course, the activities could also have a direct health component, such as learning to eat healthy foods, exercising, learning basic hygiene skills, knowing how to feed a baby better, stopping smoking, and so on. But we feel that when these direct health activities are embedded in a wider range of activities of many types, they are generally more palatable to the average person. Also, provided the principles outlined here are followed, all these activities will be health-promoting anyway. The key, then, is a wide variety of positive, attractive, well-run, popular and empowering activities that will suit all tastes in the community, and which will draw in substantial numbers of that community as participants.

4. Unity

Earlier on, when talking about diversity, we said that, from a community development perspective, a transcendent goal was a unity that took into account the diversity of a given community. This may sound like an impossible contradiction, but what it represents is both a goal and a real state of affairs that can happen when certain social and psychological conditions are met. But first we have to have it clearly seen as an overall objective.

What do we mean here? The fact that divisiveness, imbalances, internal fights and conflicts, bigotry, fragmentation and similar non-unity lead to unhappiness, hostility, destructive energy, unwellness, and many other psychological and social negatives is probably well recognized by most people. Such things are true both at the level of the human organism and at a wider social level. The transcendent aim of a community health promotion approach is, we believe, to promote both internal and external harmony, so that life enjoyment and good health are fostered through all the parts interacting together as a well-balanced whole. In particular, the "whole" we are calling a "community"—that is, a significant aggregation of people linked together by interest or geography—is of vital interest here. Such unity-in-community is also a very practical enterprise. That is, if a community can truly find out what are the deepest health and well-being aspirations of its members, even if these members are located in very disparate groupings, and truly work to meet these aspirations taking into account both the diversity and the commonality, then what we have is a whole community working together on a unified set of goals. This has the power to bring an otherwise disorganized or fragmented community together, which in turn provides that community with energy and power. We have repeatedly seen in our work how a major impact can be made, once a group of people iron out their internal differences and work in an energetic and socially supportive way on a common set of goals. This impact is not only on themselves as a community, but also on outsiders who affect their lives such as politicians and bureaucrats, and on social institutions such as government and health bodies. When there is major participation in a health promotion or community development project, and the diverse people concerned speak with one voice and really believe what they are saying with their hearts, it is a tremendously powerful social phenomenon. It can have powerful political effects, and it can have powerful effects on the participants in terms of feeling strong, effective and in control of one's life. As will be seen in Chapter 15 ("Towards a PCHP Society"), these principles can be applied to considering the structure of a new society, a "real democracy", in which community power is uppermost. Here, we just want to reiterate that a transcendent goal of PCHP is the development of personal and social strength through diverse people at the community level working together on common goals and, in so doing, having a major impact on the life of society, and on their own lives in a positive, healthy, quality of life way.

Summary

From a people perspective, participation is a vital dimension. That is, the more people involved in a health promotion endeavour at the community level, and the greater the representativeness of those people across all social groupings in that community, then the greater the impact and the strength of the processes. It is recognized that all communities contain diverse groupings, whose identities and values need to be honoured. As part of the larger community, such groupings can either operate in a mainly self-interested, detached and even conflictual way, or share in a wider, community-building and more unified approach. It is the latter we favour here as an overall goal.

L: LIFE QUALITY

The issue of quality of life (QOL) is such a central one that we devote a whole chapter to it (Chapter 4). The importance of this topic has to do with how we see the overall aims of health promotion, which we feel are not always clear to people either inside the field, or outside it. Hence we end up in confusion. Often, while a vague goal of "positive health" may be espoused, what we find in practice passing under the label of health promotion would probably better be called "prevention"—that is, the reduction of risk for, or incidence of, a given disease entity or set of such entities. We maintain that health promotion has quite distinctive goals, and that these are best characterized within a QOL context. Here we consider this issue under three headings:

1. The ultimate goal of PCHP
2. Positivity
3. Spirituality and spiritual health

The Ultimate Goal of PCHP

Without goals or clear direction, any enterprise is likely to end up not knowing where it is going, and those participating will be demoralized and confused. To some extent we see this happening at present in health promotion generally. As mentioned, although the Ottawa Charter has given many of us a valuable framework within which to view health promotion, it has also had the effect of making the area and its goals so diffuse that no one is quite sure what health promotion actually is any more. Or, alternatively, one person or group may be very sure what it is, but that view might differ quite fundamentally from that of another group also sure about what health promotion is. Like any community, the domain of health promotion is made up of quite disparate groups, coming from different disciplines, genders, ideologies, levels of professionalism, political stances, employment situations, and so on, and with different agendas according to whether one is a community worker, health educator, bureaucrat, academic, researcher, media person, or whoever. And because most of us believe in what we are doing with a passion (as distinct, maybe, from some other employment areas), then the inherent confusions and differences within the area take on an even more significant aspect.

We do not suppose what we will say here will bring the whole field of health promotion together. But in so far as PCHP represents a distinctive field within health promotion, we want to be very clear about what its overall or ultimate goals are. And these have to do with QOL. The ultimate aim of PCHP is good health within a QOL framework.

So, what does this mean? In Chapter 4, we go into this in more detail. Here, this area can be summarized by saying that QOL is largely a subjective or experiential matter that depends on how a person perceives his or her life across all the major sectors of that life. In particular, it relates to the degree to which the person is able to enjoy the possibilities that life presents to her or him.

QOL is seen as the product of a variety of determinants, both environmental and personal, and these determinants can have either a positive or negative impact. When the impact is positive, that is, the person experiences their life as positive, this experienced positivity is called "well-being". When the experience is negative, this constitutes "ill-being". Some determinants of QOL have more impact on health than on other parts of life, and it is those we are most interested in here.

Health promotion is seen as having a direct impact on health-related QOL determinants. That is, it attempts to make changes for the better in both environmental and personal factors that impact on health and well-being. The placing of health within a wider QOL context means that it is always being related to wider system factors. For example, it is clear from the model presented in Chapter 4 that many of the determinants of overall QOL will also be determinants of health, whether they be factors such as housing, social skills, physical environment, a state of peace or war, unemployment, biological inheritance, personality, or whatever. That is, on the "input" side, a wide array of factors can be considered as relevant to the "causation" of health. On the "output" side, the fact that health is seen in close conceptual proximity to other dimensions of QOL such as spirituality, community well-being, personal development, and so on means that health is inextricably tied up with these factors, and what affects one is likely to affect another. Yet we are still able to point to a distinctive entity called health, which represents that sector of QOL which interests us most in a health promotion context. "Everything is interconnected", Eastern religions tell us, and we subscribe to that view. However, such a view does not stop us focusing on a particular aspect of reality for a particular purpose. It is only when we forget the interconnections that we are in trouble.

Positivity

Implicit in many discussions of health promotion is that it is somehow a more "positive" enterprise than, say, curative medicine. That is, whereas treatment is primarily concerned with illness and the removal and alleviation of distress and symptoms, health promotion is in theory concerned more with a domain that is "beyond illness". This domain covers considerations such as states of wellness, fitness, healthiness, skill development, knowledge acquisition, supportive environments, and so on. Most of the language in this area is difficult. Terms such as "wellness", "positive health", "good health", "whole health", and so on all have slightly undesirable semantic overtones to many health promoters, yet we do not have another language to express what it is we are trying to deal with here. As someone pointed out, the English language is rich in words for negative states, and fairly impoverished when it comes to positive states. That certainly seems to be true in the area of health and medical languages.

Another reason why, in spite of pious hopes to the contrary, health promotion finds difficulty in the area of positivity, is that there is little money in it, at least in the realm of publicly funded health. (There is, of course, in many countries a profitable private sector industry related to "good health".) Although politicians, health professionals and others will often utter the words "health promotion", it is clear that what they really mean is prevention, especially if this can be related to lower costs. In short, most people will work where the money is, and the money is mainly in treatment and, to a lesser extent, in the prevention of definable diseases and problems, so that, inevitably, the best intentioned health promotion efforts get dragged in this "negative" direction. But we believe that if something *is* frankly prevention, then it is more honest to call it that, rather than to invoke the term "health promotion".

Yet another reason for weakness in the area of positivity is the inherent difficulty in measuring positive health. As a consequence, the powerful tools both of research and of data-oriented policy cannot get behind a health promotion whose focus is on positivity. And why is "positive health" so hard to grasp? The reason is mainly to do with what might be called a "narrow–broad" or a "concrete–abstract" dimension. That is, concepts like disease or illness are readily relatable to relatively narrowly defined, present or absent concrete signs and symptoms. Even these provide some difficulties in measurement, because nature is so variable, but nevertheless it is much easier to measure, say, a heart attack than it is a state of good health. In short, diseases and personal/social problems are clear, discrete, measurable entities, whereas concepts like good health, wellness, well-being and QOL are broad and vague. They simply do not have the same bite, emotional power, urgency, priority or measurability as diseases, or health and social problems like car crashes or sexual abuse.

At the same time, we believe that the sorts of life conditions that throw up many of today's diseases and "health problems" are intimately related to the issues we are talking about here in the context of positive QOL. Any lasting impact on the well-being and health of society will only come through the community, economic, environmental and personal development activities that we see as being at the heart of health promotion. And the goals to bring these about are positive rather than negative. The goals concern a better life for as many people as possible, a reasonable level of good health in society, and the enhancement of well-being, life satisfaction, happiness and "spiritual strength". Hard to measure and get funded, yes. But the whole desire to have a health promotion in pursuit of positive goals will not go away because of its difficulty. In short, with PCHP, we are firmly committed to the pursuit of positive goals in a QOL context, and believe that much of the sickness and current problems in society would disappear if we pursued these goals on a widespread basis.

Spirituality and Spiritual Health

PCHP gives an important role to the concept of spirituality, and spirituality is considered to be an aspect of QOL, as will be seen in Chapter 4. However, an argument could be made that this domain (the domain of the spiritual) concerns an area beyond that of QOL. Indeed, perhaps the ultimate goal of any true health promotion activity is not improved QOL, but something to do with the state or nature of the human spirit, soul, essence, Buddha Nature, godhead, ground of being, and so on. Concepts like empowerment and strength-building are close to some of the spiritual ideas found in many cultures, for example, the concept of *mana* or spiritual power of the New Zealand Maori, and the Chinese concept of *chi*. Even a rather vague and secular term like "human spirit" implies a nobility, strength and vitality of a special nature, which may go beyond what our concept of QOL is attempting to say. Whether or not such "spiritual" matters can be regarded as part of QOL or as goals of health promotion is a matter of debate. But, certainly, we feel that the realm of the spiritual needs attention in health promotion, and we look further at this in Chapter 8.

Summary

This section has been concerned with what is perceived to be the main goal of PCHP, which is health positively defined within a quality of life (QOL) context. QOL is seen as a subjective matter, related to the extent to which a person enjoys opportunities life presents to him or her. Health is viewed here as a subsection of a broad QOL field. The interrelatedness of health with the wider QOL field is emphasized, and many of the factors that determine overall QOL will have a strong bearing on health in this context. This goal of health promotion (good health within a QOL context) provides a positive definition, compared with prevention or other more "negatively oriented" definitions.

E: EVALUATION

The final main component of PCHP is evaluation. To some, this means an add-on, done out of a sense of duty, or in response to the requirements of a funding agency. Here, we see evaluation as a vital and intrinsic aspect of any health promotion endeavour, and as a defining aspect of an "academic" approach to health promotion. But it is not an "academic" issue as such. Rather, it is part of the honesty, self-criticism, orderliness, accountability, and desire for an optimal set of outcomes and processes, that should characterize any mature health promotion undertaking. The main beneficiaries of a well-conceptualized developmental process are not external agencies, or academics who want data for publications. They are the people themselves—those whom the health promotion endeavour is aiming to benefit. But for evaluation to be of this nature, it has to be properly thought out, built into the project from the start, and be "owned" by the community of concern. We come back to the topic of evaluation in greater detail later (see Chapter 12). Here, we would just like to emphasize the following:

1. Outcome evaluation
2. Process evaluation
3. Cybernetics and self-criticism
4. Accountability and ownership
5. The power of data

Outcome Evaluation

Outcome evaluation (as distinct from process evaluation) sometimes seems to get a bad press in health promotion. This may be because it does not capture the richness or significance of "process", and certainly an exclusive preoccupation with outcomes is probably not too healthy. However, we feel that if money, time and human effort are going into an enterprise that is believed to be valuable (and anyone working in PCHP will think this about his or her pet project), then there is a responsibility to all concerned, including oneself, to demonstrate that it has had a positive impact in health promotion terms. Also, we want to know whether it has achieved what it set out to achieve or, if not, whether it had some other kind of benefit. If the enterprise was a "failure", an outcome evaluation at least encourages one to be honest about this, and to learn lessons from what happened.

The first task of evaluation is to insist that any project is clear about its goals. The next step is to set up mechanisms from the beginning to ensure that appropriate information is collected to present evidence about whether these goals have been attained, and what other effects the project has had. Such evaluation may be quantitative or qualitative, although we favour a mix of both in most cases. The most basic kind of outcome evaluation is *goal-attainment assessment*, which is quite readily done (we discuss this later), and provides good information so long as it is honest. Such assessment refers in the first place to the overall goals of the project. However, it can also be used for the goals of any and all subprojects and activities. To this end, it is useful for all activities to have their own sets of goals around which their operation is organized.

In addition to goal-attainment information, there are a variety of other forms of outcome evaluation that can be used to get a full picture. For example, one might use *objective indices* such as available health and social measures (incidence of various health and social problems, visits to programmes, numbers of healthy children, family break-ups, crime rates, and so on). *Participation rates* in the health promotion project, and general community knowledge and impact of the project can also be assessed.

A variety of *subjective measures* are also useful, in particular health and well-being measures. Such measures aim at finding out whether people feel their health and well-being have changed as a result of their contact with the project. Closely allied to this are *satisfaction measures*, designed to find out whether people feel their personal goals were met, and how much they liked their contact with the project.

Finally, but by no means least, it is useful to have *qualitative descriptions* of the whole project process—its history, what happened, anecdotal case histories of participants' experience, and so on. In some projects, it may also be desirable to undertake this as a fully fledged "qualitative research" exercise, where, say, verbal accounts of participation or life experience are analysed fully for their context and significance.

With all these approaches, the overall aim is to make a final or periodic assessment of the overall impact of the project, notably with regard to (a) the philosophy and general aims of the project, and (b) the assessed needs of the community concerned. The point of doing an outcome evaluation is to know whether something has "worked", and has done so in a way that meets the stated philosophy, and in a way that has been to the satisfaction of the majority of those involved.

Process Evaluation

An outcome evaluation is a major and infrequent undertaking (for example, once a year for an "annual stocktaking", or at the end of a funding period). But from the beginning, we need to be collecting information that shows how we are doing, and whether we are on track. Such information serves a number of vital aspects. First, it provides vital "reinforcement" for what is being attempted—there is nothing like positive feedback to boost the morale of an enterprise, and almost all enterprises will have a more positive than negative achievement. Second, however, it will also bring errors and miscalculations to light, and no undertaking would be human without these. This is often the hardest part, because it tends to be painful and threatening to have errors and shortcomings revealed. This is why it is important to have a consensual commitment to evaluation, so that it can be conducted in an impartial and "clean" way. The consequence of revealing errors is not punishment, but a consensual working together to reset goals, or take other corrective action (see next section). The third important function of process evaluation is that it sets up a healthy climate of self-analysis and self-criticism, about which we talk in the next section as well.

At the heart of process evaluation in the PCHP approach, organized as it is around clearly stated goals, are regular review sessions (for example, weekly), where progress on all goals and subgoals is monitored. As will be seen from the examples given later in the book, this process can be done quickly, and is regarded as invaluable by those working in a project, even though it may take some effort to set up and maintain. We believe that without such internal checks, most projects will tend to float off target, and may collapse in a mess. In addition to goal reviews, other ongoing review processes are possible too, including calling in outside assessors if some activity is causing particular concern. Internally run workshops or "think tanks" on issues of staff or other concern can also be a form of useful process evaluation.

Cybernetics and Self-criticism

The term "cybernetics" comes from systems theory, and refers to systems that operate in terms of clearly defined goals or targets. That is, if one has a target clearly in mind, evaluation (especially process evaluation) serves to provide ongoing data for system correction, so that goals are optimally met. This is no more than what we were saying in the previous section, except here we are making this viewpoint quite explicit. The key to cybernetics is *continuous feedback*, which is used for ongoing correction of system activities. In a cybernetics system, "negative feedback" (i.e. feedback showing that a goal-directed system is off target) will automatically initiate self-correcting processes. "Positive feedback" confirms the system is on track. In a human system, both positive and negative feedback are essential. However, both are often overlooked or avoided for different reasons. Positive feedback, vital for morale and people's self-esteem, may be taken for granted and not made explicit. However, experience with classrooms, and almost any other collective human endeavour, shows that one cannot overlook unambiguous positive reinforcement, and those managing any human system have to build this aspect into it. As for negative feedback, no one likes this, so it tends to be avoided. The trick is to build such feedback into the system in a non-threatening and business-like way, and one way to do this is to have everyone examine "mistakes" as a problem-solving exercise, so that responsibility is shared.

Above all, an "evaluation philosophy" is one where the system is *not* threatened by self-criticism. On the contrary, the system encourages questioning at every point, with the motivation being not to criticize people (and we all make mistakes), but to enhance system performance. So evaluation means a constant asking of the question "How can we do this better?" And if something clearly is not working well, rather than feel guilty about it or otherwise punish oneself, one asks, "What can we learn from this to make it work better in the future?"

Accountability and Ownership

To the extent that a health promotion enterprise is a people or community endeavour, then there are many people with a stake in it. These people give time, energy, commitment, money, faith, goodwill, and many other valuable and personal resources. Whoever is managing the enterprise bears a responsibility to all those people to keep faith with them, and to let them know exactly what is going on. This does not mean a public soul-baring of every detail and difficulty, but it does mean an honest and sincere effort to let people know how things are going, where resources are being used, what the success is, and so on.

Therefore, any evaluation activity should be designed with this dimension in mind. Furthermore, one should be clear about how and where information is to be disseminated. Communities often get uncomfortable if the first thing they hear about themselves is from some public media source, rather than through channels closer to home. The "inner community" needs to be able to decide whether they want certain information to go further afield or not. Real efforts may have to be made through newsletters, meetings and other such means to keep the local community informed.

Issues sometimes arise relating to "who owns the information". In the past, in non-PCHP activities, especially where academics or professionals have been controlling research activities, and may be doing them for their own advancement, there has been a feeling by those being "researched" that the information does not belong to them. Also, they may feel like objects of study for someone else's benefit. Here, it is necessary to say that all research, evaluative or otherwise, should be designed and implemented in a consultatory way, with the community concerned being involved at every step. Research is generally regarded as a matter requiring special expertise, and so there is a temptation for academics and professionals to retain a non-empowering attitude with regard to it. Also, the consultation required for co-ownership of research may slow it down. And there is a risk that the proposed research will be turned down by the community, or requests will be made that the researcher does not want to meet, such as a change in design, or doing some other task for which she or he is not prepared. Regardless, these are issues that can all be faced and worked through. The main point still remains—that, at the least, research is a collaborative and "partnership" matter in PCHP. Even better, the research will be owned, controlled and perhaps even executed by the community itself (maybe with expert back-up, if this is requested). Under this model, the data and information from this research are unambiguously the property of the community, who may in turn be quite happy for an academic or professional to publish it, or otherwise use it for their own purposes, provided permission is given and people are quite clear about the intentions.

The Power of Data

In some respects, data are "mightier than the sword". That is, convincing statistics from good quality research and evaluation are very powerful, in all sorts of realms. For example, if it can be said that 80% of a community have participated in a project and, of those, 85% report significant improvements in their health since beginning participation and 90% report a high degree of satisfaction with what happened, then this is fairly convincing information for politicians, funding agencies and others who may have a strong influence on the future of endeavours. Such information also is good for the morale of those working in a project, and for the community who are supporting it or participating in it. So quite apart from all the other reasons given above for doing evaluation, data provide powerful tools for persuasion and public relations. In our experience, almost all well-done PCHP-type projects do produce impressive data, and *do work*, no matter how that is defined. To have good data to back this up is of benefit to everyone concerned.

CONCLUSION

In this chapter, we have attempted to go over the main philosophical and practical elements of PCHP. This was done by using the mnemonic "PEOPLE" to highlight the key components, namely *P*eople-centredness,

*E*mpowerment, *O*rganizational and community development, *P*articipation, *L*ife quality and *E*valuation. We saw that the central philosophical driving force is that of empowerment, which here means that the people of a community, defined as a grouping of people with actual or potential common interests, bonds and preferably geography, are in control of the enterprise, and are personally and collectively strengthened by it. The key to achieving this from an organizational point of view is the adoption of a community development approach based on the framework of organizational development, where needs assessment and clear goals are the central features. Indeed, the term "development" can be seen as being at the heart of health promotion, as distinct from other related activities such as "prevention". That is, we are aiming for constructive changes that take place relatively slowly over periods of time, but result in permanent transformations of lives, communities and environments. To do this, a high degree of participation is aimed for, and the whole undertaking is seen as being positive and strength-building. The overall aim is the enhancement of physical and mental health and well-being within a broad quality of life context. At the centre of the approach is people's everyday life experience at the community level. This approach means a different way of working than that which most professionals are accustomed to. It also means that such "expert" activities as research and evaluation are done under the control of the community to serve the interests of whatever is being done, rather than being solely to serve the interests of the professional or academic. Professionals who work in this way usually find great satisfaction in doing so, and it seldom seems to limit their activities, research or otherwise.

In Part II of this book, we return to a number of these points, and elaborate on them.

3

PLACING PCHP IN THE THEORETICAL AND POLITICAL SPECTRUM

In their critique of what they call "the new health promotion", which is characterized by concepts such as "empowerment" and "community participation", Canadian Ann Robertson and American Meredith Minkler (Robertson and Minkler, 1994) point to the fact that there are "underlying ideological conflicts, and accompanying turf battles, which have arisen in the wake of the new directions that health promotion has taken". They say:

> A fundamental ideological conflict exists about the goal of health promotion: should the goal be improved health status (individual and collective)—health as an end?; or should the goal be social justice—health as a means? Emerging from that conflict are other related ideological conflicts, including: micro-level (individual) change versus macro-level (structural) change; individual lifestyle strategies versus community-based approaches; and professional ownership versus public ownership. (p. 297)

Probably, they could have added that these conflicts are also related to where those working in the field are coming from academically, professionally and politically. Underneath much of the tension one sees in health promotion are conflicts between broad disciplinary groupings, such as the supposed "individual" and "non-structural" approach of psychology versus the sociopolitical and structural approach of, say, sociology. There are also conflicts within disciplines, such as those who support "positivist" or quantitative research as distinct from those favouring "post-modernist" or "qualitative" approaches. Indeed, there seems to be quite a lot of covert anger in health promotion, as each discipline and subdiscipline tries to stake its claim and demonstrate its superiority to the next. This is probably the inevitable result of a field that tries to be interdisciplinary.

The contradictions in the rhetoric and practice of the new health promotion have also been remarked on by New Zealand health promotion commentator Victoria Grace (Grace, 1991). For example, she says with re-gard to some of the themes of this book:

> Two years ago I completed a critical analysis of the discourse of health promo-tion in an attempt to come to terms with some of the contradictions facing me as a health promotion practitioner and researcher. One of these contradictions was particularly articulated in our specialised literature, in statements of aims and principles. It was this strong conviction among us health promotion pro-fessionals that we were empowering people, that we were developing a prac-tice that put the control with community-based people and not with "experts", that we were operating within a truly community development philosophy. I became increasingly suspicious of this noble sentiment because it seemed to me to generate a number of important contradictions. [In particular], no matter how much we wanted to position ourselves in the background, there was a strong, guiding and controlling professional agenda . . .
>   . . . I found two conflicting themes emerging from the discourse—one invol-ving providing, serving, giving, and the other involving planning, surveying, strategising, targeting, implementing, evaluating—a discourse of control. These two themes or strands were interwoven throughout people's discourse on health promotion . . . (pp. 1–2)

Our view is that the area of health promotion, and the professionals working in it, can best be viewed as a "community", in the way we concep-tualize that term here. And, as in any community, there will be a range of opinions, ideologies and agendas being represented. And there will also be a range of adherence to the "purity" of principles, such as empowerment and community development. Regardless of differences between people, com-munities can either be viewed as aggregations of subgroups who are in self-interested conflict, or be seen as entities with the potential for living harmo-niously together while acknowledging the differences between the groups and individuals concerned. Each implies quite a different underlying philosophy—one which implicitly supports anger and conflict, and the other which acknowledges difference and the presence of conflict, but tries to harmonize things notwithstanding. That is, every sector of society, even those normally regarded as "the enemy" (for whatever reason) has some-thing to offer. No group is all bad, and most operate according to their lights, even though the attribution of self-interest or other malevolent intent is very common by people who do not like another group.

With regard to the "radical versus conservative" dimension in health promotion, we (the authors) place ourselves in a conciliatory, consensus-oriented middle ground between these two poles, advocating a "just" ap-proach to health, which also (as far as possible) works with "the system", and which tries to synthesize the best and positive aspects present in all disciplines and social groupings. We realize this is a tricky place to be, and that it opens us to abuse from all sides. We will be seen as "lefties" and "radicals" by those wedded to the existing systems of "power over" and political privilege. And we will be seen as wimpish sell-outs by the politicized and aggressive left. The latter position was well put a number of years ago in the book *The Radical Therapist* (Brown et al., 1974), where it was pointed out that it was easy for a "radical" to be disconcerted by the game of "lefter than thou", meaning that no matter how "liberal" one was, there would always be a purist to the left of you making you feel like a sell-out.

In taking such a stance, we are open to the criticism of those with more "structural" leanings who may say that if we get too preoccupied with the people side of things, we will lose sight of the important social-structural problems that are oppressing people and detrimentally affecting their health and well-being. Certainly, the emphasis here is on the "people side", but it is in the context of constantly remembering the social-structural and political context. We believe it is not a case of *whether* one takes this into account, but *how*. That is, we can either adopt a health promotion stance that is "tough", political, angry and aggressive, with clear enemies and agents of societal injustice who have to be dealt with at all costs, or we can take a more conciliatory, consensus-building approach, where the aim is maximizing the power and advantage of those without power and advantage, but without an excessive siege mentality. To some extent, this comes down to a personality thing. Some people like to work in a "righteous anger" way, and others not. The issue is also related to the actual political and social situation in which one finds oneself. In countries like Canada and New Zealand, although there are clearly major social injustices and inequalities entrenched into our social systems, which are exacerbated by the current political eras of new right economics, these are not on a scale that one might find in some other countries. There may be a very strong case for radical action in some settings. But within any setting, regardless of its extremity, we believe there is a range of options about the style of working, and about the social analysis made of the situation. We are simply saying that our preference is to seek the more peaceful and conciliatory solution when this is an option.

We see that a combination of "people" and "structural" views is the best. Canadian Ron Labonte (1993) sums this position up well, when he says:

> Unless we practice thinking simultaneously in both personal and structural ways, we risk losing sight of the simultaneous reality of both. If we focus only on the individual, and only on crisis management or service delivery, we risk privatizing—rendering personal—the social and economic underpinnings to poverty and powerlessness. We may offer personally empowering services but *de facto* reinforce a structural powerlessness. But if we only focus on the structural issues, we risk ignoring the immediate pains and personal woundings of the powerless and people in crisis. (p. 57)

Certainly, one danger in taking a strong people approach is that we do respond too strongly to the immediate pressures of the "pains and personal woundings of the powerless and people in crisis". A true "developmental" health promotion approach requires us to be able to step back from reflexive "helping", to see what is needed organizationally in the medium to long term. It is important to be aware of this because our observation, from hard experience, is that those wishing to work in a health promotion way can often be swamped by the pressures to work with people in crisis situations. In order to deal with the kind of individual, group and community development we see as basic to the health promotion process, one needs to be to some extent free of the immediate pressures of crisis situations. This is not to say that we do not "care"—of course we do. But whenever possible, it is better, we believe, to have the "crises" dealt with by those whose professional roles are to deal with therapy and crisis resolution, and to have the health promoter be concerned with the more developmental side of things. Also, there is a large amount that can be done for people in crisis in the context of mutual aid and support groups, which are seen as a legitimate activity within health promotion (see Chapter 14). (However, we do not see this as "mainstream" health promotion, but on the boundary between "therapy" and "health promotion".)

The issues raised above of a personal versus a structural analysis, and the involvement of health promotion in dealing with "crises" and direct service, are central to any practical consideration of health promotion. All of us have livelihoods to pursue, and the pressures exerted by our employing agency will be a powerful determinant of what we can or cannot do. In the main, publicly funded health service agencies will put pressure on their employees to deal with the crises, rather than be engaged in longer-term development processes, and to attend to those crises in an individualistic and politically neutral way. Much of what we talk about in this book is clearly different from that, and may therefore be an ideal to which only a few currently employed health promotion workers can aspire with any sense of comprehensiveness. Yet as the case histories given later show (Chapters 12–14), it can be done.

Some similar issues arise as to the kind of "academic" or "scientific" approach we take to the health promotion enterprise. Here, we have stated that our basic approach comes from psychology, which has a strong history of positivism, individualism, reductionism and non-contextualism. To some health promoters, much of psychology is seen as "the enemy" from an academic point of view. However, like many other disciplines, psychology is changing rapidly. For example, there is currently a rapidly increasing acceptance of post-modernist and qualitative approaches within psychology, as within most other social sciences. And community psychology, which is a major force underlying PCHP as an academic area, is organized around a set of values based on empowerment, community development, cultural diversity, equity, and other key aspects of the new health promotion. No one would claim that any of this represents the mainstream of modern psychology, but it is certainly at least present within current thinking.

Although PCHP draws strongly on psychology, it is not exclusively from that territory. As will be seen in later chapters, a variety of academic sources inform PCHP, bringing in all the tools and concepts thought to be relevant to such an approach. These certainly include the analytical tools of sociology, the tradition of health education, the cultural perspectives of anthropology, and the structural and policy dimensions of political science and other "macro" study areas such as demography and geography.

In short, then, we feel it is important to be upfront about where one stands academically and ideologically. Here, we make it quite clear that we favour a middle-of-the-road approach politically—we are for change and action that betters the lives of the oppressed and disempowered, but would like to see this done as far as possible without undue acrimony, anger and aliena- tion of establishment groups. Indeed, a consensual, harmonious way of working is the one we favour, although we are realistic enough to recognize that this will not always be appropriate or possible. (And we also want to make it clear that if a "choice" has to be made between "the people" and "the establishment", then it is unambiguously the people who "win".)

Similarly, our academic stance is one which is grounded in psychology, but which draws on all relevant disciplines, and which is oriented to using any and all methodologies as appropriate. We do not hold out for either positivist or post-modernist approaches as being superior. Each has its ad- vantages and its limitations, and they need to be used as appropriate in different settings.

We acknowledge that these stances will not endear us to everyone. But at least you the reader will know where we stand.

Health promotion is currently such a large and diverse field, that no one could be expected to be all things to all people. As Labonte (1993) says in the context of the five broad spheres of empowering health promotion practice he presents, "No one professional possesses the skills (or time) to work in all five spheres". While we have no desire to present a monolithic approach to health promotion to which all should subscribe, the approach we adopt here is one which *can* be mastered by a single worker, and which at the same time provides flexibility for that person to work at a variety of levels, according to inclination, background and the demands of a given situation. PCHP pro- vides a broad, systematic approach to planning and executing health promo- tion projects at the group and community level. This approach permits the worker to move both "down" to the individual level and "up" to the popu- lation or policy level. It also provides the health promotion worker with a framework in which to work on her or his pet projects or topics, and to use his or her own specialist skills. It is, in short, an organizational framework that can be applied to almost any health promotion enterprise of a develop- mental nature, within a broad philosophical framework of empowerment, community-building and "putting people first".

II

BASIC CONCEPTS, ISSUES AND APPROACH

In Part II, we look at a selection of the basic principles covered in Chapter 2, and consider these in more depth, to provide a basic conceptual and procedural structure for PCHP. That is, rather than provide a cookbook, we would prefer that those working in the area have a broad grasp of the essential principles, and then come up with their own solutions to particular problems or situations. The overall intention of this part of the book is to stimulate a thoughtful discussion by students and others interested in general principles. However, it should be remembered that we are considering these topics in the context of PCHP, which is likely to result in different emphases than those found in a coverage of these topics in another context. Therefore, students are well advised to use standard sources on these topics (e.g. textbooks in psychology and sociology) to supplement what is presented here.

In Chapter 4, our first step is to look at what is considered to be the desired outcome of PCHP—that is, positively experienced health and well-being within a quality of life context. Then, in Chapter 5, we move on to a consideration of the most important concept in the whole enterprise—that of empowerment. Here we see that this concept sums up both a goal of PCHP (people feeling strong and in control) and the main process (people building their strength through empowering activities and organizational frameworks).

These basics are followed in Chapter 6 by outlining the approach considered the best to operationalize an empowerment-based health promotion process— that of "community development". However, although what might be called "empowering community development" provides a broad general and systematic framework for action and evaluation, we emphasize in Chapter 7 that such an approach needs to be tailored according to cultural considerations. In Chapter 8, we take a jump into territory that is usually not addressed in conventional health promotion treatises—the spiritual dimension.

Most of the concepts covered here have a history of research and thought behind them, often going back for many years, decades or even centuries. There is nothing new here, except perhaps the packaging and emphases.

4

THE OVERALL AIM OF PCHP
Health and Well-being in a Quality of Life Context

In Chapter 2, we said we felt it was very important to be clear about the aim of any health promotion enterprise. In PCHP, the aim is quite clear: it is the attainment of positively experienced health and well-being within a quality of life context.

In Chapter 2, we covered some of the basics of what this means. Here, we would like to go into this in more detail, in particular to see more exactly what is meant by the terms "quality of life", "health" and "well-being".

This we do by first looking at the concept of quality of life (QOL), basing this on a major research project in Ontario. We then argue for a concept of health and well-being nested in a QOL perspective, one which has especially to do with how "ordinary people"—the jpf's—view health.

QUALITY OF LIFE:
THE ONTARIO DISABILITY PROJECT

The issue of finding a practical, meaningful definition of "quality of life" arose in the context of a project commissioned by the Ontario Ministry of Community and Social Services, and organized through the Centre for Health Promotion (CHP) at the University of Toronto. (For short, we call it the "CHP concept".) The aim of this was "to conceptualize and design an approach to measurement as the first phase of a province-wide study of the quality of life of persons with disabilities" (Woodill et al., 1994).

This process involved getting input from a variety of sources. One was the literature on QOL in psychology, sociology and philosophy. Here it was found that, while there were many instruments designed to measure QOL, there were few attempts to look at the concept as a whole. A second, no less important, source was a series of focus groups held with people with disabilities, their families and caregivers, as well as with policy-makers. Discussions were also held with researchers working in the field of disability. In addition, there was much input from the multidisciplinary team assembled for the project, which included people with training in sociology, psychology, rehabilitation medicine, family medicine and adult education. This mix of inputs led to the development over time of a conceptual framework for QOL that is, we believe, unique in its comprehensiveness, philosophical foundation and practicality.

Although the CHP concept was developed in the context of disability, we believe it has universal application, as was its intention. To quote Woodill et al. (1994):

> The approach reported here [proceeds by] conceptualizing and measuring quality of life around the principle that people are much more alike than they are different. Human characteristics that are common to all people serve as the foundation for quality of life, while individual differences are seen as the various—and often unique—ways that individuals have of expressing these common characteristics according to their own personalities and their own environments. Therefore our approach to measuring quality of life is intended to be appropriate for all people, not only for people at various levels of developmental disability, but also for those with or without other kinds of disabilities; that is, it is a *generic* approach to quality of life. (p. 58)

It is also important to note that, since Ontario has a diverse and multicultural population, this concept has been tested across a wide variety of social and cultural groups, and has been shown to stand up well in these different contexts.

The concept of QOL arising from the CHP study is shown in Figure 4.1. (Note: the figures used here were designed by the present authors, not by the original project team. Also, the remainder of the discussion in this chapter is mainly our own. But we have used, and are extremely appreciative of, the CHP project's overall concept of QOL as a springboard for this discussion.)

Here it may be seen that QOL on the CHP model is considered to comprise nine main measurable areas, grouped into three broad categories of "Being", "Belonging" and "Becoming". The *Being* cluster covers those areas to do with people's physical, psychological and spiritual dimensions. The *Belonging* cluster has to do with people's social, living and work context and the *Becoming* cluster has to do with their work, leisure and personal development activities. Specific questionnaire measures have been developed to assess individuals singly or collectively in these areas, so this approach also has the merit of being readily quantifiable in a psychometric sense.

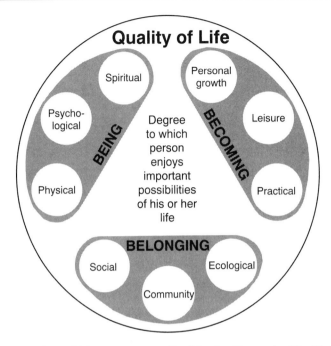

Figure 4.1: Quality of life, as conceptualized in the Centre for Health Promotion quality of life project

Each of these areas is seen as offering "possibilities" to the individual, leading to either "well-being" or "ill-being". The capacity of the person to make the most of what is offered will be a prime determinant of well-being, and this "capacity" will be a mixture of personal and environmental factors. Thus, QOL is defined as being the "degree to which a person enjoys the important possibilities of his or her life".

One important aspect of this concept of QOL has to do with *control*, and the associated dimension of *choice*. The capacity to make the most of opportunities, so that they can be enjoyed, depends to a great extent on how much control a person feels she or he has. Control has to do with autonomy (versus dependence on others), and the ability to do things. It also involves how much choice a person feels he or she has, which is in part an environmental or social matter.

To summarize, this concept of QOL is seen as a holistic one, encompassing all the main domains in a person's life. QOL is a product of how these domains are enjoyed, and this in turn is the result of the sense of control the person has in the various life situations in which he or she finds him or herself.

QUALITY OF LIFE, WELL-BEING AND HEALTH

In Figure 4.2, we see QOL is viewed as being the result of identifiable determinants, divided into environmental and personal categories. *Environmental determinants* involve both wider-system factors, impacting on but somewhat remote from the immediate and everyday control and experience of people in the community, and more immediate factors such as family, neighbourhood, workplace, school, house, community associations, and so on. The latter are close to the everyday lives and experience of ordinary people, and have the potential for at least some control at a local level. *Personal determinants* are those associated with the attributes of individuals, and are divided into two subcategories, biological and psychological. Biological determinants are aspects of the body, brain and behaviour that are relatively unchangeable. Psychological determinants represent the individual's characteristic ways of dealing with the world, which may or may not be relatively changeable.

Figure 4.2 uses the words "well-being" and "ill-being". That is, QOL determinants are able to produce both positive and negative effects.

The other point of interest in Figure 4.2 is the presence of a "feedback loop". That is, one set of determinants can interact in multiple ways with the other. For example, if the person feels a high level of social well-being as a result of health promotion efforts, she or he may then be in a position to change her or his environment, such as setting up a local support group, which then serves as a positive QOL force in that environment for many years to come.

In Figure 4.3, a further component is added to the QOL picture—that of "moderating conditions". In particular, negative determinants can be moderated by a number of variables. For example, someone might live in a chronically oppressive situation such as war, inadequate housing, no employment, high crime, etc. But if he or she feels there is some opportunity to exercise control over the situation (for example, in the war situation, joining a resistance group), then the negative QOL impact of the situation could well be changed in a more positive direction. Certainly, there is evidence from the stress literature in psychology that factors such as taking positive action or having strong social support impact positively on well-being in otherwise unpleasant situations.

In Figure 4.4, we turn our attention back to the "right-hand circle", but this time it will be noted that three of the nine components of QOL have been included in a new subfield called "health". These three components are the ones with the labels "physical", "psychological" and "social". These are the areas deemed to correspond to the three areas specified in the WHO definition of health, that is "a complete state of physical, mental and social well-being, not just the absence of disease". In spite of the controversy that has surrounded this definition over the years since it was introduced in

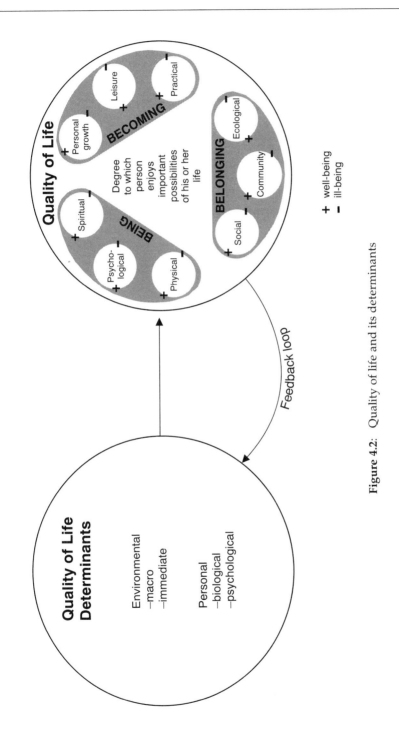

Figure 4.2: Quality of life and its determinants

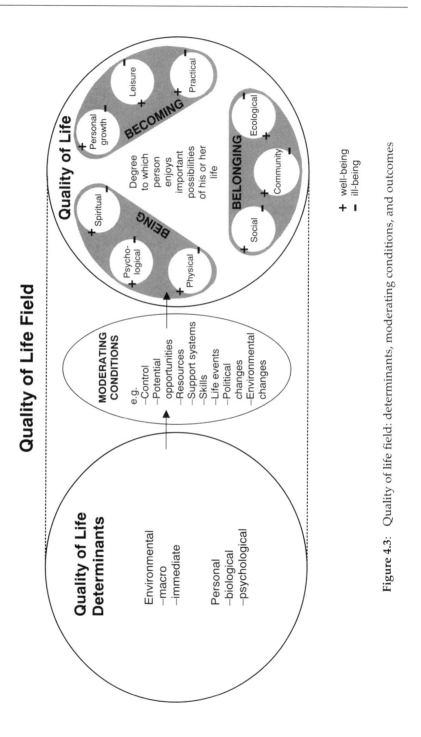

Figure 4.3: Quality of life field: determinants, moderating conditions, and outcomes

1948, it still emerges as the most frequently cited definition of health, and is the one used in the Ottawa Charter (which is the overall basis for the approach to health promotion we take here).

It could be argued that other QOL components could also be included under the term "health", especially "spiritual". However, much of the criticism over the years of the WHO definition has been that, even as it stands, it is too wide and all-encompassing (see, for example, Callahan, 1990). And, certainly, we feel it is important to try to distinguish between the terms "health" and "life" here. This has a purely pragmatic aspect to it. As economies contract, and health budgets are squeezed, an area such as health promotion is likely to lose its credibility if it is seen as trying to include "the whole of life". We feel it is wise to limit the definition of health in health promotion to an area that is unambiguous, and leave other sectors (such as welfare and justice) to deal with other issues.

In short, what we are saying here, and what is shown in Figure 4.4, is that, although "health" and "quality of life" are largely to do with the same

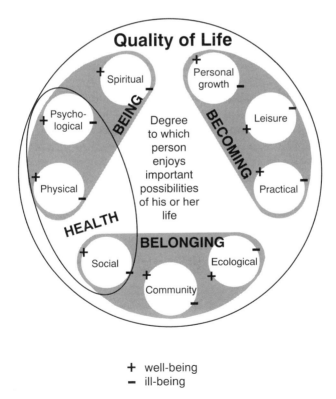

Figure 4.4:   Health as a component of quality of life

things, health is best viewed as a subfield within the QOL field. This subfield consists of the measurable "outcome" components of physical, psychological and social well-being.

In Figure 4.5, we see an amplification of the concept of the health field as a subfield within the QOL field. In the left-hand ("determinants") circle, health is seen as being affected by many or all of the same factors as affect QOL. In short, almost anything can affect health, as almost anything can affect QOL. However, because health and QOL are two different domains, each with its own set of preoccupations and emphases, we feel it is important to distinguish the health-related aspects of the overall QOL determinants from the larger array.

In summary, then, the health field is a subfield of the QOL field, but has more limited outcomes, and a different set of emphases in the areas of determinants and moderating conditions. However, the overall paradigm is the same for both. And as far as "well-being" is concerned, it refers to that dimension of the experience of life in each of the health-related QOL sectors that is regarded as positive.

QUALITY OF LIFE, HEALTH AND HEALTH PROMOTION

Figure 4.6 shows all the parts put together, and adds a set of inputs called "health promotion". As may be seen, the term "health promotion" is based on the Ottawa Charter, and the "inputs" are the five action streams outlined in the Charter. That is, health promotion as an overall entity (as distinct from that portion of it we are calling PCHP) is represented as a broad-spectrum endeavour, with dimensions ranging from the individual skills level, through community action and health service change, to wider environmental, policy and ecological concerns. Here, health promotion actions are seen as being applied to two components of the health subfield, namely the determinants circle and the moderating conditions ellipse. That is, health promotion is concerned both with the creation of an overall positive health and well-being environmental climate ("determinants"), and with specific planned interventions that have explicit health and well-being objectives ("moderating conditions").

The outcomes of health promotion will hopefully be reflected in the three health subareas of the right-hand QOL output circle. Health promotion could well involve and affect other components of that circle too, but that is not the primary interest here. The placement of the health area in a wider QOL context emphasizes the role of positive outcomes and well-being in relation to health promotion inputs. That is, health promotion would be seen not only as affecting "objective" and "subjective" components of physical,

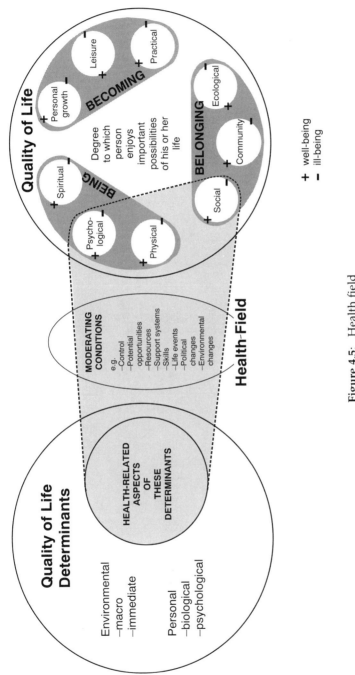

Figure 4.5: Health field

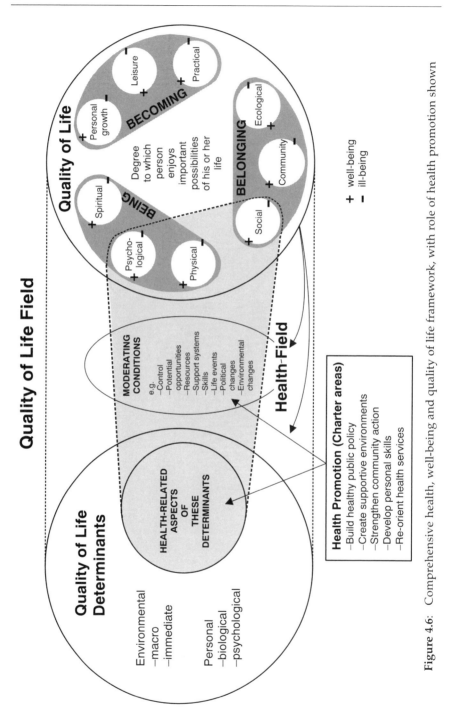

Figure 4.6: Comprehensive health, well-being and quality of life framework, with role of health promotion shown

psychological and social health as conventionally measured (which often tends to be in terms of reducing negativity such as mortality, morbidity, risk factors and "suffering"), but also as contributing generally to the positive well-being or "health-related quality of life" of people.

One final point. As we mentioned, in the Ontario research, each of the nine QOL areas has a measurement instrument associated with it, based on simple self-report. These instruments can be used with those with developmental disability, and by the rest of the population, and their usefulness has been well demonstrated. We believe that measurement instruments of this type should be included in the final outcome evaluations of any health promotion endeavour, at least for the three health subfields. We talk more about the whole area of outcome evaluation in the context of PCHP in Chapter 11.

5

EMPOWERMENT

"Empowerment" is not a word we like all that well. It is unquestionably a (if not *the*) current "buzz word" in health promotion and community development (Rissel, 1994). But like all over-used words, one can get tired of hearing it, or it tends to be misused or misunderstood.

On the other hand, there is no other term that quite captures the essence of what we are trying to say in PCHP. In PCHP, empowerment is centrally involved in both the goal and the process of what is done.

Although much has been written on the topic, there is not a great deal on the *experience* of empowerment. In general, in the health promotion literature, empowerment tends to be discussed as an abstraction, or in terms of political power structures, rather than what the *experience* of being empowered is like for people. We are not arguing for an exclusive usage of empowerment from an experiential perspective. But we are arguing for *starting* with the experiential perspective, and returning to this perspective as the centre of gravity.

In this chapter, we start with a look at "experiential empowerment", and then move on to a broader consideration of the concept of empowerment. We then discuss how this concept relates to PCHP, as an issue both of process and of outcome.

THE EXPERIENCE OF EMPOWERMENT

One striking exception to the general absence of material on the experience of empowerment is the series of Canadian studies by John Lord and colleagues of the Empowerment Research Project, Centre for Research and Education in Human Services in Kitchener, Ontario (Lord and Farlow, 1990). These studies concern what the researchers call "personal empowerment", and involve people who can clearly be identified as "disempowered" or "powerless"—those who are poor, elderly or disabled, and who have been "labelled, rejected by their communities and marginalized". The authors say:

We . . . noticed something curious—that certain individuals, in spite of the labels and extensive barriers they faced, were still able to experience a strong sense of personal control. We wondered if there was something we could learn from these individuals who had become "empowered" which might be useful to others in similar situations and to service providers. It has been suggested that the way to conduct research into empowerment is to find out how the phenomenon is actually experienced by those individual people who express the sense that they are, or are not, in control of their lives. (p. 2)

The research cited here was based on "38 people who had directly experienced the process of gaining more control in their lives". (Note that the concept of "gaining control" is what these authors put at the heart of personal empowerment.) The participants are described as covering "a range of people, including some with physical disabilities, others with developmental disabilities, women on low incomes, and a number of individuals who had first-hand experience of the mental health system".

Predictably, since participants were selected on the basis of their having gained more control over their lives, their interpretation of empowerment was, first and foremost, in these terms. For example, verbatim quotes from the subjects of the research were:

"Empowerment is the process whereby the individual feels increasingly in control of their own affairs . . . for them to be in control is a prerequisite for them to feel they can help someone else."

"The first time you conquer a fear—like getting someone to stop controlling you—you've got more confidence. The first time you can win a situation and gain more control, it's not quite so difficult next time." (p. 3)

The authors comment:

People described how little things held tremendous symbolic importance for them in terms of the enhancement of their personal control. One man with a physical disability recalled how liberating it had been for him to learn to use something as simple as a can opener; someone else had learned to cook after years of dependency. For others, their symbols related to new perceptions of themselves and their capacities: becoming involved in art after years of neglect, making plans to go back to school, finding meaningful employment, or buying a house. (p. 3)

They also say (and this is a critical comment for the approach we take in PCHP, as will become evident later):

Inherent in the perspective of our research participants was the belief that individuals should have the power to define their own needs and to act upon that understanding. Unfortunately, however, the assumption that individuals understand their own needs better than professionals is not one that is generally shared by health and social service providers.

. . . In almost all cases, something happens which leads to the person breaking out of the pattern they have been in. This often includes a strong set of dependencies, which both sides (the person and their surrounding social environment) have bought into. Many professionals and families seem to need to have others dependent on them for their own emotional gratification. And for the person concerned, it is often "easier" to be "looked after" than to suffer the pain of becoming independent. It is a vicious circle, but like all vicious circles, it can be broken. For some, it comes after a crisis or other period of difficulty, which motivates the person to do something different.

"Usually any major change, any achievement I've made has been after a time of difficulty—something that has been unpleasant or uncomfortable or just unattainable. That's when I actively go and seek change." (p. 4)

The researchers comment:

Several of our participants noted the important role played by a self-help group, a friend or colleague in accelerating their move toward personal empowerment. Another key role was that of the mentor. One woman described how a friend of hers gave her confidence in herself: "It was just her attitude . . . you know, she would say things like 'I think you're ready to have your own apartment' . . . She built up my confidence so I could say 'yes, I can do it'."
. . . A mentor or support person might be a friend, colleague, peer or service worker. In our study, such individuals were perceived as being assertive and confident, as well as accepting and valuing of the person. (p. 5)

Even more important among the social factors is participation in community activity—perhaps the single most important contribution to the development of a sense of empowerment.

Involvement in community life was mentioned by most as being key to the growth in their personal empowerment. They found that as they began taking risks and becoming more active in community life, the very fact that they were participating was itself empowering. (p. 4)

Lord and Farlow's summary comment on the role of participation is illuminating, and goes to the heart of the community and personal empowerment process from a "people perspective"—the valuing of people as people, as full, worthwhile human beings:

When we began our research on empowerment we assumed that as people gained increasing control in their lives, they would inevitably wish to channel their energy into consumer activist groups working for structural or policy change. What we found, in fact, was that regardless of the nature of the participation—whether it was based on common recreational or cultural interests, political concerns, or the desire for mutual support—simply being accepted as a member of the group was an important factor for many people.

The collective is where individuals find a network in which they establish a level of trust and comfort with others. Their involvement is based on their ability to contribute at that point in time, and on their commitment to group goals. One requirement for empowerment seems to be the feeling of being valued for whatever one can contribute, no matter how small it may be. As some of our participants noted, it is this sense of being valued, together with the initial act of participation, that leads the person to gradually assume more responsibility within the group or organization. This, in a sense, is true community participation. (p. 7)

EMPOWERMENT AS SEEN BY COMMUNITY PSYCHOLOGY

Community psychology is unique in the field of psychology for subscribing to a clear set of values. Of these values, "empowerment" has always been at the top of the list. In community psychology, we have an academic discipline virtually built around the concept of empowerment. Therefore, we would like to present the community psychology view of empowerment here. To do this, we draw on the perspective of Julian Rappaport of the University of Illinois at Champaign, one of the key figures in the development of community psychology as a field.

Rappaport says that "community psychology has had the character of a social movement", and comments that to "the extent that a discipline becomes more a profession and less a social movement, its practitioners are likely to become more defensive, conservative, and lose their sense of urgency" (Rappaport, 1981). He goes on to say:

To hold on to urgency requires a cause that transcends ourselves, one that holds symbolic power. To burn with fervour for some higher purpose, be it expressed in understanding or in action, is to be alive and to push ourselves to create the possibilities for change. The most important contributions from community psychology have been fuelled with a sense of urgency. To give up such urgency is to live with mediocrity. (p. 8)

Empowerment, then, as the premium value of community psychology, lives within this atmosphere of social movement, a higher purpose, a sense of urgency, and aliveness. Indeed, the same sense tends to pervade the area of health promotion, which is probably why so many of us feel passionate about it, and why a concept like empowerment tends to provide a rallying point for those who are "alive" in their health promotion work. In short, "empowerment" in this context takes on quite a different quality from that just discussed in the Ontario study, although it too shares elements of this special human flavour.

As part of an important social movement in the latter part of the 20th century, Rappaport (1981) puts the empowerment issue into this context:

We are witnessing the rise of the idea of rights over needs. The paradox for the remaining years of this century will be encapsulated in a struggle between opposing views of the poor, the physically disabled, the mental patient, the retarded person, the juvenile, the elderly, and so on, as dependent persons to be helped, socialized, trained, given skills, and have their illnesses prevented, or as citizens to be assured of rights and choices. Symbols and imagery will be very important in this struggle. It makes a great deal of difference if you are viewed as a child or as a citizen, since if you believe it you are likely to act the part . . . and if those in power believe it they are likely to develop programs, plans, and structures that will help you to believe it. (p. 11)

Here, Rappaport has some important words to say about prevention, which reinforce our own view that health promotion has to be seen as a separate enterprise from prevention, even though the two are typically confused.

[Under the prevention model], the crucial element of "expert/helper", or the "doctor/patient relationship", or at least the "student/teacher relationship", will be maintained. There will be no question about who is "up" and who is "down". Even programs aimed at so-called structural change, when framed in terms of "prevention", create a metaphor that despite intentions, when adopted by our social institutions yields all the wrong symbols, images, and meta messages . . .

Prevention programs aimed at so-called high-risk populations, especially programs under the auspices of established social institutions, can easily become a new arena for colonization, where people are forced to consume our goods and services, thereby providing us [the professionals] with jobs and money. (pp. 12–13)

Rappaport then goes on to say:

Many of us have placed our bets on the ideology of prevention. It is my contention that this ideology has outlived its usefulness and is one-sided at its core. It is a product of our failed social history and it creates the wrong symbolism . . . I will make the case that empowerment rather than prevention is far more promising both as a plan of action and as a symbolic ideology for the social movement called community psychology. [He could just as well have said "health promotion"!]

By empowerment I mean that our aim should be to enhance the possibilities for people to control their own lives. If this is our aim then we will necessarily find ourselves questioning both our public policy and our role relationship to dependent people. We will not be able to settle for a public policy which limits us to programs we design, operate, or package for social agencies to use on people, because it will require that the form and the meta communications as well as the content be consistent with empowerment. We will, should we take empowerment seriously, no longer be able to see people as simply children in need or as only citizens with rights, but rather as full human beings who have both rights and needs. We will confront the paradox that even the people most incompetent, in need, and apparently unable to function, require, just as you and I do, more rather than less control over their own lives; and that fostering more control does not necessarily mean ignoring them. Empowerment presses a different set of metaphors upon us . . .

Empowerment implies that many competencies are already present or at least possible, given niches and opportunities. Prevention implies experts fixing the independent variables to make the dependent variables come out right. Empowerment implies that what you see as poor functioning is a result of social structure and lack of resources which make it impossible for the existing competencies to operate. It implies that in those cases where new competencies need to be learned, they are best learned in a context of living life rather than in artificial programs where everyone, including the person learning, knows that it is really the expert who is in charge . . .

Empowerment lends itself to the possibility of a variety of locally rather than centrally controlled solutions, which in turn fosters solutions based on different assumptions in different places, settings, and neighbourhoods . . . Rather than a top down or forward mapping of social policy it is a bottom up or backward mapping that starts with people and works backwards to tell officials what social policies and programs are necessary . . . This means that empowerment will not only look different depending on what sort of problems in living one is confronting, but it may even look different in each setting that it operates. Diversity of form rather than homogeneity of form should dominate if the operating process is empowerment . . . (pp. 12–17)

Rappaport goes on to identify the principal location for the implementation of an "empowerment ideology" as he calls it:

The implications of an empowerment ideology force us to pay attention to the mediating structures of society, i.e., those that stand between the large impersonal social institutions and individual alienated people . . . These include the family, the neighbourhood, the church, and voluntary organizations. These are the places where people live out their lives, and the more control they have over them the better . . .

It is now quite obvious that for many people their network of friends, neighbours, church relationships, and so on, provide not only support, but genuine niches and opportunities for personal development. How can we learn to help to create new settings, or to assist those who are isolated from such settings or those who are trapped in settings which are harmful rather than helpful, if we do not spend a great deal of time observing, describing, and collaborating? (p. 19)

These excerpts from Rappaport (1981) provide what might be called the context or philosophy of empowerment, in which a sense of personal empowerment can be fostered. That is, we need to adopt whole new ways of looking at people in society, especially in relation to what are conventionally labelled as "problems", and our professional work needs to be directed by this. Rappaport calls this an "empowerment ideology", and elsewhere he refers to the "empowerment social agenda" (Rappaport, 1992). We feel that "health promotion" and "community psychology" are interchangeable here, at least in the framework of PCHP.

EXPERIENTIAL EMPOWERMENT: A DEVELOPMENTAL PERSPECTIVE

In this section, we return to the theme of empowerment as an experience. As Lord and Farlow (1990) showed in their research, empowerment is a developmental process that evolves over time. An understanding of this aspect of empowerment is, we believe, critical to any health promotion work based in the empowerment concept. This dimension of development in empowerment has perhaps been articulated most clearly in a classic treatise by community psychologist Charles Kieffer, of the University of Michigan at Ann Arbor. We now turn to this. Kieffer's paper, published in 1984, was called "Citizen empowerment: A developmental perspective". In this, Kieffer charted the course of 15 intensively studied individuals through their involvement in grass-roots community action programmes, most of which had a political aspect, and documented their personal development process over four or so years. A clear pattern of "personal empowerment" emerged that was common to all. This is how the group of participants was described:

> Fifteen participants were included in the study. All participants had emerged through activity in "grassroots organizations" which were citizen-initiated, pragmatically oriented, and community-based. Selection was limited to those who had become active in the latter 1970s. Each was characterized by (1) self-acknowledgement of personal transformation, (2) recognizable transition into proactive and multi-issue engagement, and (3) evidence of continuing commitment to involvement in local political processes or grassroots leadership roles. They were all identified through networking with formal leaders in regional advocacy and training organizations.
>
> Of this sample, five were male and ten were female—a fairly typical proportion of gender distribution in community organizations. Ages ranged from thirty to sixty-five. While most had not moved beyond a high school diploma, two had recently completed Bachelor's degrees, and one had attained a Master's degree in nursing. One was a migrant labourer, two came from Spanish Harlem, four were residents of ethnic, working-class neighbourhoods in the Northeast and Midwest, four were from communities in the Central Appalachians, and four were from southern agrarian and industrial areas. Typical of the individuals involved were a working-class mother who had become the prime force in constructing a community health clinic, a migrant labourer who had become an organizer and boycott coordinator, a former junkie and gang leader who had become a leader in an urban homesteading program, and a retired labourer leading efforts against brown lung disease. (p. 13)

These participants, as can be seen, were selected on the basis of their having recognizably become "empowered" over a period of time. Therefore, they may well be unusual people, about whom it is difficult to make generalizations. Also, in so far as the participants were involved in "political" activities and had developed a political consciousness, they are not necessarily typical of those who are in more "benign" health promotion activities, although some of these will have a political edge as well. Notwithstanding these reservations, our experience is that most of those participating in community health promotion activities, and getting into those in a meaningful way, experience some elements of what is described here to a greater or lesser degree. What *is* striking about the people studied by Kieffer is how clearly they illustrate the strength of *participation* as a force in producing a sense of personal empowerment. And, as we have emphasized above, the attainment of this "health" is through a gradual *development* process, rather than something that happens in response to an isolated intervention or event, even though such things may *trigger* a subsequent development process.

The key aspect of the "empowerment" that Kieffer documents is not so much the concept of "control", as we have seen so far (although that is there too), but something he calls "participatory competence":

> How *do* individuals manage to move beyond . . . situations of powerlessness and oppression? In what ways do the shared experiences of a scattered group of individuals illuminate the elusive idea of empowerment? What emerges from their lengthy and detailed retrospection is a common and consistent conception of empowerment as a process of becoming as an ordered and progressive development of participatory skills and political understandings. Empowerment then assumes a dual meaning. It refers both to a longitudinal dynamic of development and to attainment of a set of insights and abilities best characterized as "participatory competence". (pp. 17–18)

The first thing that emerges from Kieffer's research is that all participants, like those in the Ontario study, had experienced a strong sense of powerlessness in their lives. However, unlike the Ontario participants, this was less associated with a clearly identified source of disempowerment like a disability, than with a more general existential powerlessness, arising out of the social and cultural milieu in which they lived. Kieffer says:

> In sum, the sense of powerlessness is viewed as a construction of continuous interaction between the person and his/her environment. It combines an attitude of self-blame, a sense of generalized distrust, a feeling of alienation from resources for social influence, an experience of disenfranchisement and economic vulnerability, and a sense of hopelessness in socio-political struggle. (p. 16)

Each of the participants in the study was then seen to move through a clearly definable developmental process of four stages, about which Kieffer comments:

> While this research sought to illuminate empowering transitions as processes of development, I had never anticipated the consistency and clarity of the developmental model which ultimately emerged. (p. 26)

The developmental process takes considerable time and involvement on the part of the participants:

> Empowerment is inescapably labor-intensive. For all these participants, at least four years of intensive experience underlies attainment of enduring commitment. (p. 27)

So what then are the four "eras" or stages of development that produce "a fully mature participatory competence" (for which read "empowerment", as defined in the context of this group of people)? Kieffer defines them as follows:

Stage 1: The Era of Entry

This happens when people with an already well-developed sense of community and "integrity" decide to respond to "tangible and direct threats to individual or familial self-interests".

Stage 2: The Era of Advancement

Here, the key elements are contact with a "mentor" or significant other person (cf. the Ontario study), and social support from peers involved in the same enterprise.

Stage 3: The Era of Incorporation

This is where participants settle down into a full level of activity within the context in which they are operating. (Note that all these people are "participants" in some organized community project, which is how we see empowerment as best happening in PCHP.)

Stage 4: The Era of Commitment

Now the skills and competencies are well established, and are being incorporated into the person's life generally, and into new undertakings. A whole new range of values, self-concepts, skills and sense of self-worth have become integrated into the person's way of dealing with the world. "Many", says Kieffer, "transpose their capacities into new careers helping others. Some commit themselves to more traditional political roles. All have committed themselves to adapting their recent empowerment to continue proactive community mobilization and leadership." At this stage, their experience means that they are capable of leadership and the sharing of knowledge and skills with others.

The conclusions that Kieffer draws about the nature of empowerment in this community development context is close to our understanding of that term as it applies in PCHP.

> [In the light of this study], empowerment can be viewed as an attainment of an abiding set of commitments and capabilities which can be referred to as "participatory competence". This state of being and ability incorporates three major intersecting aspects or dimensions: (a) development of more positive self-concept, or sense of self-competence, (b) construction of more critical or analytical understanding of the surrounding social and political environment, and (c) cultivation of individual and collective resources for social and political action. It is important to emphasize that these are interconnected elements of a unitary notion of socio-political competence . . .
>
> The fundamental empowering transformation, then, is in the transition from sense of self as helpless victim to acceptance of self as assertive and efficacious citizen. Achieving empowerment also implies developing the skills and resources needed to confront the root sources which create and perpetuate victimization. (pp. 31–32)

EMPOWERMENT: A STRUCTURAL PERSPECTIVE

Up to now, we have focused on empowerment primarily as an experiential phenomenon—that is, as something that people actually feel, actually experience in a psychological sense. We have seen that central to this conception of empowerment are psychological elements to do with *control* (the sense that I can influence the course of events rather than have events totally control "me"), with *competence* (yes, I can do this and do it well), with *self-esteem* (I am valued for what I am and what I can do, and I believe in myself), with *contribution* (I feel I have knowledge, skills and confidence I can pass on to others) and, above all, with *participation* (I have moved beyond "me" into a wider, valuable collective enterprise). The overall effect seems to be a sense of "real power" and strength in the world, which in time leads on to making an impact and contribution. These psychological components of a sense of empowerment develop through a *realistic* history—that is, doubts about oneself transform into these more positive feelings and beliefs as it becomes clear that one *does* have a degree of control, one *is* competent, one *is* valued, one genuinely *does* have something to contribute, and one *is* part of a "larger cause". As we have seen, at the heart of empowerment is a developmental process, often taking a long period, maybe years, to grow to significant levels. However, many academic representations of empowerment do not have this quality about them. Empowerment seems a more abstract entity having to do with a commodity called "power". Very often, the question is how people can "possess" this power (rather than develop it), and this is often seen as a matter of "taking" power from those who already have it. This in turn makes empowerment closely allied to a conflictual or political agenda. Certainly, the question of empowerment often does arise in a political context, particularly where there is obvious political or bureaucratic oppression.

At this point, we will take the more "structuralist" perspective of the well-known Canadian health promotion teacher and commentator Ron Labonte, and outline some of its main points. Labonte is far from being an "extreme" structuralist, and he acknowledges the need to synthesize "psychological" perspectives with broader political and structural elements. But he certainly takes a more structural view generally than that represented so far in this chapter, and so we will use his approach to outline a more structural perspective on empowerment.

Labonte says that at the heart of empowerment is the word "power", meaning "the ability or capacity to act or perform effectively, to exercise power" (*American Heritage Dictionary*, 1973, quoted in Labonte, 1990). He points out that the verb "to empower" can be used both transitively and intransitively. Transitively, it means bestowing power on others. Intransitively, it means "to gain or assume power" (*The Concise Oxford Dictionary*, 1971, quoted ibid.).

Labonte states:

> Empowerment exists at 3 levels: intrapersonally, it is the experience of a potent sense of self, enhancing self-esteem and self-efficacy; interpersonally, it is the construction of knowledge and social analysis based upon personal and shared experiences; and, within communities, it is the cultivation of resources for personal and sociopolitical gains. (1993, p. 65)

He also breaks empowerment down another way, in terms of the kind of professional practice involved in fostering empowerment. This is represented as an empowerment continuum, with five "nodes" consisting of personal care, small group development, community organization, coalition building and advocacy, and political action (Labonte 1990, 1993). He represents these as an "Empowerment Holosphere" made up of overlapping subspheres. Of these, he says:

> While the Empowerment Holosphere links actions around all five spheres, no one professional possesses the skills (or time) to work in all five spheres. The Holosphere represents an imperative for the organization as a totality . . . The point of the Holosphere is to make clear the professional and organizational necessity to seek (identify, nurture) linkages between these different social levels of action. (1993, p. 56)

At the *personal care* level, Labonte is mainly concerned with those *services* which provide "case care" to clients or individual people in the community. How does one work in an empowering way here? The key to this is what is called "developmental casework", in which an explicit goal [is] the development (empowerment) of the individual receiving the support, and the creation of links between those individuals . . . This approach builds towards community organizing and coalition advocacy—and hence the political elements of empowerment and the structural level remain explicit . . . (p. 57)

The second component of the Empowerment Holosphere is *small group development*. Labonte clearly feels that the small group is the key social-structural unit for both empowerment and community process:

"Community" is often represented as the engine of health promotion, the vehicle of empowerment. But it may be more accurate to say that the *small group* is that locus of change, that vehicle of emancipation. "At the level of the small group, society has always been able to cohere" (Homans 1950, p. 468). Nations rise and fall, institutions come and go, civilizations flourish and perish, even community organizations wax and wane, but one ineluctable aspect of humanity is its formation into small groups. To understand the *group* and its dynamics is to understand an essence of what is human. The group is where we forge our identities. The group is where we create our purpose. Only in interacting with others do we gain those healthful characteristics essential to empowerment: control, capacity, coherence and connectedness (Wallerstein 1992). (1993, p. 58)

The third component of the Empowerment Holosphere is *community organization*.

Community organization describes the process of organizing people around problems or issues that are larger than group members' own immediate concerns. (1993, p. 61)

According to Labonte, this area inevitably raises the issue of conflict:

Conflict within and between communities is a fact of life. Many relatively powerless groups only create their identity as a community in opposition to or conflict with those groups or communities that are more powerful than themselves. This dynamic has been at the base of all Alinsky-style organizing efforts, and has been successfully used to create communities from the seemingly intractable conditions of isolation and apathy. (1993, p. 61)

The fourth subsphere of the Holosphere is that of *coalition building and advocacy*, which Labonte describes as "tonics to the limitations of community organizing". The two terms are defined as follows:

Coalitions are groups of people with a shared goal and some awareness that "united we stand, divided we fall"; advocacy means "taking a position on an issue", initiating actions in a deliberate attempt to influence private and public policy choices. The two are linked in the Holosphere because advocacy usually involves coalitions.

. . . There are two differing facets of advocacy. First, professionals themselves can increase the strength of their own political voices, taking positions on such broad healthy public policy issues as social welfare reform, housing needs or affordability, employment policies, environmental standards or any other concerns that may be expressed by individual clients or by community groups of clients. Second, professionals can aid community groups in their own advocacy by offering knowledge, analytical skills, information on how the political and bureaucratic structures function and so on. (1993, p. 69)

The final component of the Labonte Holosphere is called *political action*. This is seen as an extension of coalition building and advocacy.

The line between what comprises coalition advocacy and what constitutes political action is fuzzy; one important difference may lie in the role played by organizations and groups loosely considered to be representative of social movements. A coalition or alliance of groups coalesces action around a particular issue that cuts across differing commonwealths of values; a social movement brings its commonwealth of values to multiple issues. (1993, p. 71)

The essential aspect of action at this wider political level is the necessity for collaboration between people and groups. This in turn relates back to the perennial issue of intergroup conflict, and how one transcends that.

That intergroup conflict is both healthy and perhaps essential to social change should not lead us to shun the necessity of uniting diverse, conflicting groups at some higher level of community. Community-as-ideal, the moral or spiritual resonance of the word, is what gives it both its power and its appeal. As Gardner (1991) expressed, pluralism without commitment to the common good is pluralism gone berserk. Pragmatically, the community born in conflict or struggle rarely survives the eventual peace "unless those involved create the institutional arrangements and non-crisis bonding experiences that carry them through the year-in-year-out tests of community functioning". (1993, pp. 72–73)

EMPOWERMENT IN A PCHP CONTEXT

By now, the reader will hopefully have some "feel" for empowerment, and how we interpret it in a PCHP context. In this final section, we would like to make that more explicit.

First and foremost, empowerment is to do with an inner experience of personal strength, effectiveness and power. This experience is closely allied to "health", and has to do with a body–mind–spirit condition of wellness, confidence, wisdom and being fully alive. But as well as being an inner experience, it is also something that others can quite clearly "see" that a person has "got"—empowered people have a sense about them of groundedness, quiet confidence and inner strength. They are also likely to be helpful and skilled. And although this may describe the "fully empowered" person, there are many grades between disempowerment (the absence of these things) and full empowerment. In conventional psychological terms, the person has a discernible level of competence, self-esteem, confidence and self-efficacy, and feels in control of what is going on in his or her life. Empowerment may refer to a limited number of situations, or it can be present across most or all of the life situations in which a person finds her or himself.

Second, although this empowerment is in the first place an inner and experienced state, it is brought about to a large degree through social determinants, and has an important social impact. That is, empowerment comes about typically in people who initially feel disempowered, either personally or environmentally. A change is then triggered through some event (which may be a crisis or external threat), and the path toward empowerment is then typically assisted by a "mentor" or other strong person, whose attributes and belief in the person are such that the person is inspired to take action to change either his or her own or the environmental situation. Usually, the "path" to empowerment is in the context of a social group engaged in an enterprise of relevance to the person, and which offers the potential for the person to develop new skills and competencies and to be valued by others for that. As these skills and competencies develop, the person is in a position to be socially effective, to help others, to take political action, to serve as a mentor to newcomers, and so on.

Third, as suggested here, the stages in this empowerment process follow a fairly predictable developmental course, which may take a considerable period of time and be marked by conflict and barriers, but which ultimately leads to the growth of "personal power" in that person. Our observation is that while this may take years for some people, for others it can happen in a matter of weeks, although no one is ever fully "empowered", and there is always room to develop.

Fourth, since much disempowerment is associated with social and environmental conditions that are oppressive or otherwise disadvantageous to the people living in them, then frequently the activities associated with empowerment have a political or "fight the system" aspect to them. In such situations, there are bureaucratic, political, industrial or other major power bodies who are seen as self-interested, oppressive or conservative in their actions, and become a potential or actual "enemy". In these cases, empowerment-related activity will most likely have a "political" or "conflictual" edge to it, requiring very assertive action.

Fifth, community process and development is intimately involved in our concept of empowerment, because of the fact that most empowerment comes about as a product of, to use Kieffer's term, participatory competence. That is, it is *participation* in a group or community activity that is central to empowerment as we see it here. Disempowerment is often experienced most acutely at the social group level of personal, family and local community life, and the "solutions" are also best handled, at least initially, at this level. (Participation is obviously tied up with the quality of life concept of "belonging", as well as of "becoming".) Also, there exists in most empowering processes a sense not just of benefiting oneself, but also of working towards a more general common good. As we become more confident and efficacious, we are simply less self-preoccupied, and there seems to be a deep sense in most people of the value of contributing for the wider community good. Thus, the commitment of people to extend their skills and efficacy to contribute to a more general "community benefit" is a typical part of this process. (This is perhaps more to do with the "being" aspect of quality of life.)

Sixth, as pointed out by Rappaport, Labonte and others, empowerment is a term that applies at a variety of people levels (personal, interpersonal, community), and at a variety of societal levels (group, community, coalition, political, etc.). Empowerment can be viewed personally or structurally, and it becomes an issue whenever power is an issue, and where power imbalances exist. Here, there are two different points to be made. One is that it may be somewhat confusing to assume we are using exactly the same concepts when talking about these different levels of empowerment. Power at the personal level, for example, may be quite different from power at the institutional level. In particular, there is confusion about the concept of power as a commodity that can only be traded by subtracting from the power of one person or group to add to the power of another, and the concept of power as a developmental thing, which is available to all. Here, we recognize that power issues and imbalances apply at all levels, and that our aim should be one of "equity", where we are working to bring resources and power to those who are clearly under-resourced and disempowered. But ultimately our interest here is in the development of personal empowerment, which we see not only as of direct benefit to health, but also as equipping people to take the political and advocacy action necessary to change the systems within which they live.

Seventh, and finally, this view of empowerment has a direct impact on how we, as professionals, interact with people at the community level. One can take a cautiously empowering approach, and work within the constraints of one's employing body, trying to be as "empowering" as that situation will allow. Or one can be "radically" empowering, and aim at full community self-determination and control. As Rappaport points out, we constantly have to be scrutinizing what our employers allow us to do, and what we ourselves do, to determine the extent to which our work is genuinely empowering.

To conclude then, PCHP is concerned first and foremost with a radical empowerment—that is, one where the people are unambiguously in control and self-determining. Such empowerment is fostered through developmental processes, which lead in turn to a direct experience of personal power by the people concerned. These developmental processes will take time, and will occur at three main "people" levels—personal, group and community. We believe the most potent level at which to work is that of community, which allows us to be oriented both "up" to the larger systems of society, and "down" to the intimate and personal. The key to working in a community empowerment way is through organizational approaches within the community that foster the developmental processes we have alluded to, and which provide the opportunity for the "participatory competence" that is at the heart of the kind of empowerment we are concerned with here.

6

COMMUNITY DEVELOPMENT

At the beginning of the last chapter, we noted that "empowerment" was a currently fashionable word in health promotion. Likewise, the term "community development" is also fashionable. According to Robertson and Minkler (1994) in their critique of "the new health promotion movement", the central features of this movement have to do with empowerment and community dimensions, and this view is echoed in a variety of places. However, like "empowerment", terms such as "community participation" and "community development" mean different things to different people, and the real meanings often get obscured.

This chapter is primarily about "community development". However, the way we use the term may not be how others see it. What we would like to do here is to study the concept of community development as it relates to PCHP.

At the heart of this analysis of community development is the concept of *development*. We start by looking at what this means.

DEVELOPMENT AS A CONCEPT

The term "development" has to do with a gradual growth or evolution towards a full, more mature, or better state. *The Concise Oxford Dictionary* (1984) says that development is a "gradual unfolding, fuller working out; . . . growth; evolution . . .; full-grown state; stage of advancement", and that "develop" as a verb means "to unfold, reveal or be revealed, bring or come from latent to active or visible state; make or become known; make or become fuller, more elaborate or systematic, or bigger; . . . make progress; . . . come or bring to maturity".

It is often hard to make much sense of dictionary definitions, but there are some key points here, and we will return to some of these. One is that the changes associated with development tend to be *gradual* and *evolutionary*, rather than being a single or circumscribed event.

A second feature of development, as defined by the dictionary, is that it tends to arise from, or be an enhancement or realization of, *latent potentials that are already present.* So often, as professionals, we feel that we have to "add" something to a person or community to make them "better". However, a developmental viewpoint requires something that is often very difficult for professionals to feel, and that is a basic *trust* in the wisdom, good sense, motivation and potential of ordinary people. The ordinary person, unspoiled by academic and professional input, is often much wiser than professionals are about what is appropriate for his or her life, and the life of the community in which she or he lives.

A third aspect of "development" is a sense that there is a movement toward something that is better, healthier, fuller and more desirable. This is clearly the assumption behind our use of the word here. Also, there is a sense of things becoming both more orderly and more elaborate in this process.

Finally, and connected to the last point, there is an overtone of "systematic" to the concept of development ("make or become fuller, more elaborate or systematic, or bigger"). This is also a very important point. The trick is getting the right balance between "structures" and "systems" to ensure that things develop in a fruitful way, but also to ensure that there is the encouragement of spontaneity, enjoyment and creativity.

COMMUNITY DEVELOPMENT: HISTORICAL AND CONCEPTUAL DIMENSIONS

In PCHP, we see community development as having to do primarily with the development of a sense of community and community cohesion. However, like "empowerment", there is a whole domain of *political* discourse about community development. Furthermore, the term "community development" is applied in many sectors outside health, and in developing countries it often has a predominantly economic dimension. We look at this briefly here through a discussion by Ian Shirley (1982), Professor of Social Policy at Massey University, New Zealand.

Shirley puts community development into a broad sociopolitical context, by regarding it as part of the history of "human settlements", and of the overall economic structure of rich and poor actions, and the rich and poor in individual countries. He sees the concept of "development" in terms of that proposed by Max Weber (1946), as having to do with the question "What shall we do and how shall we live?" To show how complex and wide ranging this issue is, Shirley writes of the word "development" (as used in the term "community development"):

> Cognitive and linguistic dissidence is evident in the very definition of "development". Freyssinet (1966) lists over 300 alternative interpretations. These

definitions differ in space, from country to country and region to region; they differ in time, from stage to stage, and from civilisation to civilisation; they differ according to goals, standards and values. Seers (1972) for example, sees development as a synonym for "improvement" but what do we mean by improvement? Does it mean an increase in material living standards, the transformation from an agrarian to an industrialised society, or is improvement synonymous with the equal distribution of resources, power and status? Whose development are we talking about, for what ends and by what means? (p. 13)

From the perspective adopted in this passage, "development" is seen as occurring at many different levels, in particular, at the level of the individual, the institutions responsible for values and norms (including family and tribe), and the State (especially in its "planning").

As far as "community development" (as distinct from just "development") is concerned, Shirley sees this as deriving from three main sources. First there is the obvious disparity between rich and poor nations, the latter being collectively referred to as "the Third World", "the South", or "underdeveloped" countries, which are characterized by "mass illiteracy, a traditional outlook on life, low levels of health and housing, and widespread despondency". Here, the desire for "development" at the community level is clearly part of the overall wish of people to better their lives at the local level.

Second, in industrial and "post-industrial" societies, there is general dissatisfaction with "increasingly impersonal and remote government apparatus". Here, presumably, there is a wish to bring more power back to the local and "personal" level, and for local people to "develop" their own living situations in ways they feel are under their control.

Third, community development has arisen from "the discovery and visibility of poverty in so-called affluent societies, coupled with a new pride among minority groups in their own cultural identity, and the vocal even militant insistence of many groups that they should participate in decision making processes that affect them". In short, there are many subgroupings or "communities" in our societies who want a better life and more power for themselves, and this is seen as a development matter.

In the same book, McCreary and Shirley (1982) discuss the history of development ideologies. They describe the interaction of colonizing nations with "underdeveloped" territories in the 19th and 20th centuries, and hold the position that the aim of the colonists was mainly to "modernize" these settings to suit their economic and cultural interests. Half a century or so ago, the key to this was seen to be education.

In the 1940s education was identified as the way to make sense of the world and the means by which colonial territories might be developed. Mass education, *education en base*, and fundamental education, were all terms used as synonymous for development. Confronted with technological innovations in the Western world and an apparent resistance to change within the Third World, administrators, and in particular those in the newly formed United Nations, latched onto community development as an educational enterprise. (pp. 36–37)

This ideology continued through the 1950s, with many colonial governments setting up conferences, "clearing houses", programmes and other endeavours to promote this view of community development.

McCreary and Shirley tell us that, by the 1950s, there had also developed an "applied anthropology" related to community development. Its emphasis was especially on the linkages of Western technology with development, although there was also a feeling of "social responsibility" about this. Out of this developed "a theory of community development", of which features were:

- Concern with the general wellbeing of the "community" as opposed to any sectional or special interest group.
- A commitment to activities based on principles of self-help and the active participation of members of the community.
- The articulation of programme objectives and processes defined by the community, as opposed to any programme imposition from outside.
- The recognition and acceptance of supplementary technical advice and material assistance from some external agency.

These elements were adopted by community agencies such as the United Nations, and in this incorporation community development became "a process designed to create conditions of economic and social progress for the whole community with its active participation and the fullest possible reliance on the community initiative". (p. 41)

In the 1960s and 70s, we came to an era that McCreary and Shirley characterize as "The Rediscovery of Poverty". That is, it became clear that within the so-called "affluent" countries, a substantial portion of the population were living in totally unacceptable conditions in terms of income, housing, health, basic rights, and quality of life generally. One aspect of this era was the principle of maximum feasible participation of residents, the areas, and members of the groups served.

This . . . provision [maximum feasible participation] resulted in a bitter struggle for power, and when the concept of citizen participation modelled on community development in under-developed areas was applied in the political climate and civil rights movement of the mid-1960s it created "an explosive mixture and was interpreted by some as a call to revolution". (p. 44)

McCreary and Shirley feel that this approach was an advance in so far as it tended to be sensitive to the local "culture" of communities, and the poverty groups within them, and thereby reflected the "anthropological" approach mentioned previously. However, they say that there was not a serious structural analysis, and the all-important power and institutional structures leading to poverty were not really addressed.

They point out that, when this approach failed to have any appreciable impact on "adequate shelter, full employment, or services and amenities to the poor", the focus shifted to lifestyles and a broader cultural perspective, which moves us into the health promotion era, beginning in the mid-1970s. It is probably true to say that, since then, "community development" as a major movement and philosophy has largely faded, and is often regarded now as "old hat", being something that is not relevant in a modern age of monetarism, the market place and mass communication. However, we hope it is clear that we, the authors, feel that a return to a community development perspective, on an "empowerment agenda", is what health promotion (and the world) now needs.

THE "HEALTH EDUCATION" MODEL OF COMMUNITY DEVELOPMENT

The foregoing discussion of the history and concepts of community development was from a general economic and societal perspective, without specific reference to health. However, throughout much of the period we have been talking about, there was a distinctive community health-related development approach. For want of a better way of designating it, we will call this the "health education" approach, largely because it is most strongly associated with the discipline of health education, especially as this was manifested in its American form. However, the approach is wider than health education as such (and is also not especially "educational" in the classic meaning of that term), and versions may be found in the community mental health movement, in community psychology, in organizational development, and other areas. Indeed, it underlies the approach we discussed earlier as "organizational development", and is the direct ancestor of the PCHP approach to community development we advocate here.

In the US, the terms "community organization" and "community development" are frequently used synonymously. In practice, however, they often mean slightly different things. "Community organization" is, in some respects, the broader term, and means a variety of methods, issues and ideologies involving community action in association with professional input. "Community development" tends to mean that aspect of community organization where the concerns are more with longer term development of typically, but not necessarily, a locality-based community. Certainly, it is the latter usage we incline towards here.

A good idea of the interchangeability of the two terms, and how they fit with American health education, is given in a paper by Emma Carr Bivins called "Community organization—an old but reliable health education technique", published in 1979 in *The Handbook of Health Education*. Bivins identifies this approach to health education as having come out of the 1940s and 50s, "the formative years of the profession" (Bivins, 1979).

> Among the grassroots approaches that continue to be productive is community organization, in the fullest and most classical sense of that term. For a while, the community organization process was ignored, and, in some quarters, repudiated. However, community organization—or community development, as some prefer to call it—may be experiencing a revival. This is all to the good. As far as a number of proven practitioners are concerned, community organization is at the very heart of our mission.
>
> Perhaps one reason why community organization had been held in low regard was a fallacious assumption that the process is applicable only to small communities and rural areas, not to big cities and complex ghetto areas. [However], community organization really fits both rural and urban settings. (p. 110)

One of the hallmarks of what is sometimes called "community health education", of which the matters we are talking about here are a part, is that it involves a systematic planning process, with needs assessment, clear goal-setting and evaluation. This is well illustrated by Dignan and Carr's (1981) book *Introduction to Program Planning: A Basic Text for Community Health Education*. This outline shows its age in terms of its somewhat experts-know-best, lifestyle approach. The concept of empowerment is not present, and the authors speak of "services", "planning for individuals, groups and systems", and health education programmes which are to be "targeted" at population groups to get them to behave in healthy ways. Notwithstanding these shortcomings, the type of systematic, planned approach espoused by these health educationalists has value as a broad structure. If the details in what follows are not studied too closely, the framework provides a general approach not unlike the one we adopt as a general organizational model in PCHP, with adaptations, of course, to make it under full community control and to make it "empowering".

Dignan and Carr outline three broad aspects to a planned approach:

> Program planning can be considered as part of an administrative cycle involving three phases: program planning, program implementation, and program evaluation. These three phases intertwine naturally, and in the ideal situation, should function to influence program outcomes. Program outcomes are the products of the activities included in the program, their quality, appropriateness to the needs of the population, and effectiveness. Program planning is the phase in which the details are planned for the delivery of the service in question.

The implementation phase is the period of time when the program plans are "tried out". . . .

The program evaluation phase is when the outcomes of the program are measured. Are the outcomes the same as stipulated in the program plan? The evaluation phase may also include a review of how the processes of planning and implementation proceeded. Process evaluation adds a broader view of what has taken place through consideration of such issues as time and re-sources required, and the efficiency of the planning group's actions. (p. 6)

In 1985, a chapter by Breckon et al. (1985) called "Using community organization concepts", in the first edition* of their book *Community Health Education*, shows a "modern" concept of community development akin to the grass-roots, community-controlled, empowerment model we advocate here. According to these authors:

Community organization involves helping a specific group or subgroup of people organize for action. It also becomes apparent that the concept is essen-tially process oriented rather than task oriented, in that once the community is organized, many tasks can be accomplished and problems solved.

Accordingly, a widely accepted and time tested definition by Ross [Ross, 1967] states that "community organization is a process by which a community identifies its needs or objectives, ranks these needs or objectives, develops the confidence and will to work at these objectives, finds the resources (internal and external) and in so doing, extends and develops cooperative and collab-orative attitudes and practices in the community".

The definition presupposes the importance of the community in that the com-munity decides which tasks need to be done and the order of their priority. Likewise, the community not only identifies resources and cooperatively accom-plishes the task, but more importantly also extends and develops collaborative attitudes and practices in the community . . . [This] suggests that the most effective and lasting change comes from within a group and is largely handled internally.

Community organization skills [of the health education professional], then, involve methods of intervention whereby a community is helped to engage in planned, collective action. They are efforts to mobilize the people who are affected by a community problem. They are part of the process of strengthen-ing a community through participation and integration of the disadvantaged and other subgroups.

The extent of consumer involvement varies considerably, leading Arnstein (1969) to conclude that structures organized to facilitate community participa-tion are, in reality, forms of manipulation, tokenism, placation, or consultation. Arnstein sees partnership, delegated power, and citizen control at the other end of a continuum illustrating degrees of community participation. Com-munity organizers are generally committed to some form of citizen control but recognize that often a partnership between members of the community and government authorities is necessary to improve the economic and social condi-tions of communities. (pp. 101–102)

---

* The third edition of this book in 1994 has essentially the same passage. We quote from the 1985 edition to illustrate the historical progression of thinking. We thank Donald Breckon for allowing us to quote from the 1985 edition. A fourth edition is due in 1998.

Breckon et al. make explicit reference to the concept of empowerment:

Another tenet of community organization concepts is the orientation towards power. As suggested earlier, this principle holds that power should reside in the community and that the process is, in large part, empowering the community to act. This process requires analysis of the power structure of a community, with power being defined as the ability to either block or induce change. Many sources of power and influence exist, including political position, control of information, knowledge and expertise, social standing, and money and credit. Knowing that power may be "possessed but not expressed", that is, used only when necessary, is important. If the premise is accepted that change usually produces conflict, then power struggles are inevitable. An understanding of the nature of power and of where and in what degree it exists is an important ingredient in helping a community engage in planned change. (pp. 102–104)

Health Community groups should remember that (1) large numbers are power, (2) coalitions are power, (3) a unified position is power, (4) members who are in credible positions are power, (5) voting is power, and (6) money is power. (pp. 106–107)

The approach advocated by Breckon et al. emphasizes community control, empowerment, facilitation by the organizers, and good organization. These are also the basic principles of PCHP. Although they were presented here as appearing in health education only in the mid-1980s, it is clear from the writings of Ross (1955, 1967) and Arnstein (1969) that these ideas were around much earlier.

According to Meredith Minkler, Professor of Health Education at Berkeley University, these community organization concepts date back, at least in America, to the 19th century. In the 1990 book *Health Behavior and Health Education*, she contributes a chapter called "Improving health through community organization" (Minkler, 1990). In this, she provides an overview of a modern community organizational approach within health education, while also looking at the historical origins. We close this section of the chapter with a look at what she says.

Unlike the other outlines mentioned so far, Minkler puts the concept of empowerment right at the forefront of the approach. She begins by defining "community organization" as:

the process by which community groups are helped to identify common problems or goals, mobilize resources, and in other ways develop and implement strategies for reaching the goals they have set. (p. 257)

She goes on to say:

Implicit in this definition is the concept of empowerment, viewed as an enabling process through which individuals or communities take control over their lives and their environment (Rappaport, 1984). (p. 257)

And:

> Strict definitions of community organization also suggest that the needs or problems around which community groups are organized must be identified by the community itself, not by an outside organization or change agent. (p. 257)

In looking at the history of community organization, which Minkler does almost entirely from an American perspective, it seems important to note that "community organization" (and, for that matter, "community development" as was discussed earlier) does not have its origins in the health field as such, but has come from more general political, economic and social welfare arenas. In the US, the professional usage of the term seems to have come from social work, but the phenomenon itself was preceded by a more political, grass-roots history.

> The term *community organization* was coined by American social workers in the late 1800s in reference to a specific field of activity in which they were engaged. This was the period of history marked by the mushrooming of charity organizations and settlement houses for new immigrants and the poor, and "community organizing" was the phrase used to describe social workers' efforts to coordinate services for these various groups (Mowat, 1961; Garvin and Cox, 1987) . . .
> . . . Several important milestones in the history of community organization took place well before and outside of social work and related fields. These antecedent and concurrent developments include such occurrences as the post-Reconstruction period organization of blacks by blacks in this country, to try to salvage newly won rights that were rapidly slipping away. The Populist movement in the American South, which began as an agrarian revolution and became a multisectoral coalition and a major political force, was also an important contributor, as was the labor movement of the 1930s and 1940s, which taught the value of forming coalitions around issues, the importance of full-time professional organizers, and the use of conflict as a means of bringing about change (Garvin and Cox, 1987). (pp. 258–259)

In the 1940s, there was said to be a "new vision" of social work, "as a means of helping people change, not merely adjust to, the *status quo*". Then in 1955 was published the classic textbook on community organization practice, *Community Organization: Theory and Principles*, by the previously mentioned Ross. The book was an important influence in promoting the "new vision", and represented, says Minkler, "the concept of a professional organizer as a change agent working 'with' rather than 'on' communities".

Another important influence in the 1950s and 60s was that of Saul Alinsky, the famed American community organizer. According to Minkler, whereas Ross's approach (like our own) "stressed methods of consensus and cooperation", Alinsky "stressed confrontation and other conflict strategies", which Minkler describes as "equally valid—and often more useful—approaches to social change". Alinsky worked with "white ethnic workers" in an area of Chicago, and was directly concerned with power issues. Minkler says that Alinsky was especially notable for his recommended process of "disorganizing" a community before it can be "organized", and then following this by pursuing winnable targets.

> Alinsky stressed the need for "disorganizing" communities before they can be organized (stirring discontent, creating a dissatisfaction with the status quo); identifying and "freezing" targets that are winnable, specific, and local; and using nonviolent conflict to build community-wide identification and participation (Alinsky, 1972). (p. 259)

Other important influences were the civil rights movements of the 1950s and 60s, notably the black rights activities of Martin Luther King and others, followed by organizational efforts associated with the women's movement, the gay rights movement, and the anti-Vietnam War movement. These were followed by the anti-poverty programmes alluded to earlier, and their principles of "maximum possible participation" (even though Minkler notes these typically resulted in "maximum feasible misunderstanding"). Minkler also mentions international developments in the 1970s and 80s, notably those associated with the WHO and Unesco. She singles out the 1978 Alma Ata Declaration on primary health care for special mention, saying that it "was heralded as a turning point in the international health field, in part for giving new meaning and emphasis to the role of community organization and participation in health". In short, the Alma Ata Declaration was one of the first international documents to make the specific link between community organization/development and health, even though, at this stage, it was mainly in the context of "health care" and "health services", rather than health promotion. (The 1986 Ottawa Charter for Health Promotion makes specific reference to its parentage in the Alma Ata Declaration.)

Minkler then goes on to a discussion of the meaning of "community", and makes what is probably the most important new point for our discussion here. She says, quite rightly, that how we conceptualize "community" will have a major influence on how we go about our community organizational or community development work.

As is mentioned in almost all discussions of community, at least in the health context, there are two broad ways of characterizing it—one that is largely geographical, and the other that is largely "interest" or "specific group" based. This is, in fact, a very important division, and one that often underlies much tension in the community development field.

According to Minkler,

> While typically viewed in geographical terms, communities may also be non-locality identified and based instead on shared interests or characteristics, such as ethnicity, sexual orientation, or occupation (Fellin, 1987) . . . (pp. 261–262)

She then cites Fellin (1987), in the book *The Competent Community*, as identifying "two types of theories relevant to the concept of community":

> The first of these, the ecological system perspective, is particularly useful in the study of geographic communities, focusing as it does on population characteristics such as size, density, and heterogeneity, the physical environment, the social organization or structure of the community, and the technological forces impacting upon it . . .
>
> In contrast, the social systems perspective focuses primarily on the formal organizations that operate within a given community, exploring the interactions of community subsystems (economic, political, and so on) both horizontally within the community and vertically as they relate to other, extra-community systems . . . (p. 262)

Minkler goes on to discuss different models of community organization, and bases this discussion on the well-known typology developed by Rothman and Tropman (1987).

The Rothman and Tropman system basically divides community organization practice into three models: locality development, social planning and social action. Of the first of these, locality development, Minkler says:

> Locality development is a heavily process-oriented model, stressing consensus and cooperation and building group identity and a sense of community. (p. 263)

This category is closest to what we talk about in PCHP. The concern is with self-help, community capacity and integration, the emphasis is on democratic processes and land-based generic community, and the basic strategies involve a "broad cross-section of people involved in determining and solving their own problems". The basis of this is consensus and community people discussing issues with each other. The professional or community organizer works as a facilitator or "enabler-catalyst", and the aim is to share and develop skills on the part of as many community people as possible.

Although what Rothman and Tropman call "locality development" is the dominant model we adopt, it is by no means an exclusive categorization. Elements of the other two models are also needed. Of these models, Minkler says:

> By contrast [to locality development], social planning is heavily task oriented and stresses rational–empirical problem-solving—usually by an outside expert—as a means of ameliorating or solving selected problems. In Rothman and Tropman's words (1987, p. 94), the concern in social planning "is with establishing, arranging and delivering goods to people who need them. Building community capacity or fostering radical or fundamental social change does not play a central part".

The third model, social change, is both task and process oriented. It is concerned with increasing the problem-solving ability of the community and with achieving concrete changes to redress imbalances of power and privilege between an oppressed or disadvantaged group and the larger society. (pp. 263, 266)

Minkler says that, across the different approaches to community organization, there are a number of principles that can be seen as central. These are as follows:

1. Empowerment

From the community organization perspective, Minkler sees empowerment as happening on two levels. The first is "individual-level empowerment through involvement in community organizing", which occurs as the result of such psychological factors as social support and a generalized sense of control or "coherence" (Antonovsky, 1979). The second she characterizes as "community-level empowerment, operationalized in part as increased community competence", the topic of the next principle.

2. Community Competence

This she sees as having to do with the different groups in a community collaborating successfully in identifying their needs, goals and priorities, and in deciding on and implementing the action required to meet these (Israel, 1985). Two practical aspects of achieving this are seen to do with "social network techniques", whereby the social ties and groupings in a community are identified and strengthened, and "leadership development", which involves local people being "animators", "facilitators" and other such community organizational roles (Hope and Timmel, 1984).

3. Participation and "Starting Where the People are At"

Within a health education context, "participation" is seen as analogous to the principle of active rather than passive participation in the learning process, or "learning by doing", which has been an especially important principle in adult education.

As for "starting where the people are at", this is identified as "perhaps the most fundamental tenet of health education practice". In particular, this involves the health educator, as change agent, beginning with people's "felt needs and concerns rather than with a personal or agency agenda". Minkler says, "Only when issues are selected by the community itself can a real sense of 'ownership' emerge, and this sense of ownership of the organization is critical to empowerment and to the ultimate development of competent communities."

4. Issue Selection

By this, Minkler is referring to those "needs", "wishes", and "felt" matters which will provide rallying points for community action. It is necessary, she says, to distinguish between "problems", defined as "things that are troubling", and "issues", defined as "problems that the community feels strongly about" (Miller, 1985). Important here are the methods used to gather the information on which to base goals. As Minkler says, "Nominal group process (Delbecq, Van De Ven and Gustafson, 1975), door-to-door surveys, and the use of Freire's (1972) problem-solving ideological methods may all be effective for this purpose."

5. Creating "Critical Consciousness"

This principle refers to the concept of "conscientization" deriving from Freire (1972), one of the most influential figures in modern health education at the community level. Freire and the teachers he trained worked with groups of oppressed, illiterate peasants in South America, teaching them to read, and also to analyse their own situation from a political and social perspective. "This method stressed a relationship of equality and mutual respect between group members or 'learner-teachers' and the facilitators or 'teacher-learners' who engaged them in problem-solving dialogue designed to help them elucidate the root causes of problems they had identified."

This overview given by Minkler of the community organization enterprise is the closest so far to how we see the community development process in PCHP. In particular, her emphasis on community control, self-determination, and genuine empowerment through active involvement in every aspect of the process is what we feel the enterprise is about.

COMMUNITY DEVELOPMENT IN DEVELOPING COUNTRIES

We have emphasized before that the "bottom line" for an empowering community development approach in health promotion is "community control". Some of the best examples of community control in the community development context come from the Third World. In a 1989 issue of the *Utne Reader*, a report by Worldwatch researcher Alan Durning is excerpted, and we would like to quote from this here (Durning, 1989). Called "Grass roots groups are our best hope for global prosperity and ecology", this article shows both the power and the prevalence of grass-roots community development action around the world. It involves literally tens of millions of people, and is in a rapid phase of growth, much of it in response to the major environmental threats (such as deforestation) happening in many areas.

Many of the groups involved are illiterate and impoverished, with little or no conventional political power. Yet their determination, their organization and their courage mean that "big powers" such as governments and major corporations are listening, and often positive social, health, environmental and political effects result from these activities, sometimes in a fundamental way.

Durning clearly feels that grass-roots groups are a world force to be reckoned with. After describing the economic, social, political and environmental factors endangering communities around the world, he says:

> In the face of such enormous threats, isolated grass roots organizing efforts appear minuscule—10 women plant trees on a roadside, a local union strikes for a non-toxic workplace, an old man teaches neighbourhood children to read—but when added together, their impact has the potential to reshape the earth. Indeed, local activists form a front line in the world wide struggle to end poverty and environmental destruction. (p. 40)

> These groups cover a wide variety of activities, including workplace co-ops, suburban parents committees, peasant farmers unions, religious study groups, neighbourhood action federations, tribal nations, and innumerable others. Although widely diverse in origins, these groups share a common capacity to utilize local knowledge and resources, to respond to problems rapidly and creatively, and to maintain the flexibility necessary to adapt to changing circumstances. (p. 41)

For the most part, these groups arise because of threat or disruption to established ways of life, something that is occurring in many locations around the world.

> Grass roots action is on the rise everywhere, from Eastern Europe's industrial heartland, where fledgling environmental movements are demanding that human health no longer be sacrificed for economic growth, to the Himalayan foothills, where multitudes of Indian villagers are organized to protect and afforest barren slopes. As environmental decay accelerates in industrial regions, local communities are organizing in growing numbers to protect themselves from chemical wastes, industrial pollution, and nuclear power installations. Meanwhile in developing countries, deepening poverty combined with often catastrophic ecological degradation has led to the proliferation of grass-roots self-help movements.
>
> In the third world, especially, traditional tribal, village, and religious organizations—first disturbed by European colonialism—have been stretched and often dismantled by the great cultural upheavals of the 20th century: rapid population growth, urbanization, the advent of modern technology, and the spread of Western commercialism. Community groups have been formed in many places to meet the economic and social needs these ties once fulfilled.
>
> In the face of seemingly insurmountable problems, community groups around the planet have been able to accomplish phenomenal things. (p. 42)

The following are just three of the many examples of what has been done.

In Lima's El Salvador district, Peruvians have planted a half-million trees; built 26 schools, 150 day-care centres, and 300 community kitchens; and trained hundreds of door-to-door health workers. Despite the extreme poverty of the district's inhabitants and a population that has shot up to 300,000, illiteracy has fallen to 3 percent, one of the lowest rates in Latin America—and infant mortality is 40 percent below the national average. The ingredients of success have been a vast network of women's groups and the neighbourhood association's democratic administrative structure, which extends down to representatives on each block. (p. 42)

The world's most acclaimed community forest movement, Chipko, shows how grass-roots action to defend a resource can grow into far more. Born in the Garhwal hills of Uttar Pradesh, India, Chipko first drew fame for its sheer courage. In March 1973, as a timber company headed for the woods above one impoverished village, desperate local men, women, and children rushed ahead of them to *chipko* (literally, "hug" or "cling to") the trees, daring the loggers to let the axes fall on their backs.

Since its initial success, the movement has deepened its ecological understanding and . . . has gone beyond resource protection to ecological management, restoration, and what members call "eco-development". The women who first guarded trees against loggers now plant trees, build soil-retention walls, and prepare village forestry plans. (p. 45)

An African federation popularly known as Naam is among the most successful of the world's grass-roots movements at mobilizing people to protect and restore natural resources in an area degraded from overuse. Building on pre-colonial self-help traditions, Naam taps vast stores of peasant knowledge, creativity, and energy to loosen the grip of poverty and ecological deterioration in the drought-prone Sahel region of West Africa. With origins in Burkina Faso, it now spills over under different names into Mauritania, Senegal, Mali, Niger, and Togo.

Each year during the dry season, thousands of Naam undertake projects chosen and designed *with minimal assistance from outsiders* [our emphasis]. Along with five neighbouring communities, for example, the settlement of Somiaga built a large dam and a series of check dams to trap drinking and irrigation water and to slow soil erosion. Villagers piled caged rocks by hand to form a dam four meters high and 180 meters long. Meanwhile, hundreds of Naam farmers have adopted a simple technique of soil and water conservation developed by Oxfam-UK, in which stones are piled in low rows along the contour to hold back the runoff from torrential rains. While halting soil loss, these dignettes increase crop yields dramatically. (p. 45)

While the community control element is clear in these examples, especially the last two, Durning acknowledges that the optimal situation is often where there is cooperation between government and community:

The greatest obstacle to community action is that communities cannot do it alone. Small may be beautiful, but it can also be insignificant . . .

The largest challenge in reversing global ecological and economic deterioration is to forge an alliance between local groups and national governments. Only governments have the resources and authority to create the conditions for full-scale grass-roots mobilization. In the rare cases where national–local alliances have been forged, extraordinary gains have followed. South Korea and China have used village-level organizations to plant enormous expanses of trees, implement national population policies, and boost agricultural production. Zimbabwe has trained more than 500 community-selected family planners to improve maternal and child health and control population growth. In the year after the 1979 Nicaraguan revolution, a massive literacy campaign sent 90 000 volunteers into the countryside; in one year, they raised literacy from 50 to 87 percent. Even under Ferdinand Marcos' repressive rule in the Philippines, the National Irrigation Administration amazingly transformed itself into a people-centred institution, cooperating with peasant associations. (p. 48)

Of course, it may be that even many national governments are "small" compared with some of the forces in the world today.

The prospects for grass-roots progress against poverty are further limited in a world economy in which vested interests are deeply entrenched and power is concentrated in a few nations. Thus reforms at the international level are as important as those in the village. (p. 48)

This discussion of grass-roots community organization and power may seem remote from the settings with which many of our readers will be familiar. However, there is no reason why "grass-roots power", meaning "community control", cannot be operative in any community. Certainly, there are examples of many developed countries having well-formed community-controlled groups, often mobilized around environmental issues.

Environmental issues and grass-roots politics play a major role in the new nationalist movements rocking the USSR . . .
    In those regions where nuclear power is still on a growth course—Japan, France, and Eastern Europe—anti-nuclear movements have grown dramatically since the 1986 explosion at Chernobyl . . .
    In Western industrial nations, community-based organizations set their sights on everything from local waste recycling to international trade and debt issues. The ascent of the German Green Party in the early '80s was partly a product of an evolution in this movement from local to national concerns . . .
    Paralleling a steady rise in neighbourhood organizing on local social and economic issues, the U.S. environmental movement experienced a marked grass-roots expansion in the early '80s. Local concerns focus particularly on toxic waste management, groundwater protection, and solid waste problems. (pp. 47–48)

Community-controlled community development activities are not just limited to environmental concerns. The community psychology and other literature has many examples of neighbourhood and other community projects that show these principles in action. To conclude here, we would like to quote from another *Utne Reader* article in the same issue, which illustrates well what a community-controlled, grass-roots community development project can do.

This article is excerpted from the Chicago Community Renewal Society's *Occasional Papers* (Boyte, 1989), and as the title suggests ("People power transforms a St Louis housing project"), the project is mainly to do with housing and living environment. But it also has a lot to do with health, well-being and quality of life.

Bertha Gilkey lives today in Cochran Gardens, a St. Louis public housing project featuring flower-lined paths, trees and grass, play equipment for children, a beautiful and clean neighbourhood, happy and trusting people. Gilkey grew up in the very same housing project when it was an ugly urban scar filled with broken windows, graffiti, rubbish, frequent shootings (both kinds), angry and fearful people. The change is one of the most dramatic stories dealing with government housing in our lifetime. And there might well have been no change at all except for Bertha Gilkey—and her hard, astute community organizing.

As a teenager she attended tenant meetings at a nearby church, and when she was 20 years old, Bertha was elected by the Cochran residents to chair their tenants' association. Since that time, the project has not been the same. Bertha had both short-range and long-range strategies, but she told me that she dared not tell anybody about the long-range strategy. Nobody would have believed her.

Bertha and her group started with small things. What did people really want? What could actually be done? Everyone wanted a laundromat again. All the project's previous ones had been vandalized . . .

The laundromat was a success. Next, the group organized to paint the hallways, floor by floor. "Everybody who lived on a floor was responsible for painting that floor," says Gilkey. "If you didn't paint that floor, it didn't happen . . . The elderly who couldn't paint prepared lunch, so they could feel like they were a part of it, too."

While sprucing up the physical appearance of their building, Bertha and her organized tenants reintroduced a kind of conduct code for their unit. A committee established rules of behavior and elected monitors on each floor. No fights, no garbage out the windows, no loud disruptions, etc. Slowly people got the message. People got involved. Living conditions improved, bit by bit.

They renamed their building the Dr. Martin Luther King Jr. Building. Symbols were important. "Everything we did, we had a party and a celebration," Gilkey says. "There would be a dedication for everything." Even the new laundromat had a ribbon-cutting.

Reaching the young people was another of Gilkey's key strategies. Changes were initiated in schools. "Kids wrote papers on 'What I like about living here', playing up the positive . . . Gradually, in an indirect way, we were rebuilding self-esteem, telling the kids it's all right to live in public housing."

Today Cochran Gardens high-rises are completely renovated. There is a community centre, courtyards, tennis courts, playgrounds, and the Cochran

Plaza town houses, built to reduce density in the complex . . . Other [associated] ventures include a catering service, health clinics, day-care centres, and a vocational training program. After showing me through Cochran Gardens, Bertha Gilkey asked rhetorically, "Isn't this beautiful? Isn't this the way poor people are supposed to live?"

How did all this happen? A lot of work, a lot of dedication, a lot of years. A lot of organizing. Gilkey sums it up: "Either you plan or they plan for you."

As I finished my visit to Cochran Gardens, Gilkey turned to me and said, smiling, "This goes against the grain, doesn't it? Poor people are to be managed. What we've done is cut through all the bullshit and said it doesn't take all that. People with degrees and credentials got us in this mess. All it takes is some basic skills."

I asked her about the principles that have created a success at Cochran: self-help, dignity, empowerment, responsibility. Are these transferable to any community? "Yes, yes," she smiled. "If we can do it in public housing, it can happen anywhere." (pp. 46–47)

If this passage were being read by a class in community development and health promotion, then it would be a good basis for a discussion. What were the key elements here? Are these transferable to other settings? Is it translatable into a health promotion context? Is it, in fact, health promotion?

One issue needs comment here. In true American style, the role of a single person, Bertha Gilkey, is played up. This raises the question—is a single charismatic person like Bertha essential for the success of a project like this? Certainly, Bertha appears to have been the "secret ingredient" for the superb transformation that took place in Cochran Gardens. Our own experience is that the key leaders in any community development enterprise do have to be special people, with a blend of people skills and organizational skills—a rare but not impossible mix. Almost any community has its Bertha Gilkeys. What PCHP is about is setting up a framework that is likely to find the Berthas, make their life easier, and also bring in the whole community in a way that does not rely on one person's unique charisma. Leaders come and leaders go. They are crucial. But any project that relies on a single person is doomed to fail. The aim is generic people power, where in any community the Berthas are identified and supported, and others are on their way to empowerment and leadership.

The Third World and Cochran Gardens stories are vivid models for what can be done. Many professionals are sceptical—it is natural, because such community-controlled endeavours do not fit readily into the way most professionals have been trained to work. Professionals still have a vital role to play, a topic we return to later in the book. But we hope enough has been said here to show the central role of community development in any PCHP consideration, to demonstrate the necessity for radical empowerment and community control, and to support our assertion that, even in a modern, fragmented society, a true grass-roots approach is possible.

7

CULTURAL DIMENSIONS

In health promotion, the two areas we have just discussed—empowerment and community development—have been recognized as having an important role by many of those working in the field. Now we want to turn to two less familiar areas—culture and "spiritual" aspects of health. In this chapter, we look at the cultural dimension, and in Chapter 8, the spiritual.

To put this discussion in perspective, we need to recall what PCHP is about. Health promotion that is not PCHP ("non-PCHP") is about policies, broad views of populations, top-down decisions, interventions designed to make people change their habits, and a scientific view that regards people as "subjects" or "statistics" to be studied in an "objective" manner from the outside. PCHP, on the other hand, is concerned with the actual experience of people, typically in groups, and nested in their everyday living environments. The aim is the empowerment and enhanced health, well-being and quality of life of these people on their own terms, and in a developmental, strength-building context.

Both non-PCHP and PCHP are aware of such matters as "culture" and "social class". However, in non-PCHP, these are largely matters for classification in terms of demographic variables, with perhaps some interest in the "cultural differences" between people. In PCHP, what we are interested in is how people of different cultures view the world, and also how we, as professionals, relate to people of other cultures in a way that respects these world views. In this context, "empowerment" relates to the development of strengths and personal power in ways that enhance and value existing cultural systems.

As with the other topics we have covered, we are not concerned with an exhaustive overview of the area. Rather, what we want to do is get an understanding of the importance of culture from the perspective of PCHP. And it *is* important. Since PCHP starts from an experiential perspective, we first have a look at culture from an experiential point of view.

CULTURE FROM AN EXPERIENTIAL PERSPECTIVE

Since this book is being written by a New Zealander and a Canadian, we will try, as far as possible, to make the cultural discussion relevant to those settings. However, the aim is also to demonstrate the universals.

New Zealand has a total population of under four million, and the dominant cultures are English-speaking European (often called by the Maori term *Pakeha*) and Maori, the indigenous people (who refer to themselves as the *tangata whenua*, or "people of the land"). The Maori population is about 13% of the total. (Although Maori have a strong and distinctive culture, there has been so much intermarriage in the 200 or so years of European settlement, that there are now no "pure-blooded" Maori left.) In common with many countries, New Zealand has experienced a "cultural revolution" in the past 20 years, as Maori (who have had one of the fastest birthrates in the world) have asserted their culture, after a century or more of legal and social injustice, the legacy of colonization. At the heart of this are issues of land, as they are with so many indigenous people who have been colonized. Also at issue is the preservation and status of the language, as well as many other aspects of the rich and "spiritual" Maori culture. New Zealand now recognizes itself as a "bicultural" country, with two main races, and many of the land injustices are currently being worked on, guided by the Treaty of Waitangi, signed in 1840 as a covenant between the Maori and the British crown, guaranteeing Maori continued sovereignty over their land and sea domains, in return for becoming British citizens.

However, New Zealand is not just "bicultural". It is also "multicultural". There is a substantial migrant population, chief among whom are Polynesians from South Pacific island countries, notably Western Samoa, Tonga, the Cook Islands, Tokelau and Niue. (Auckland, the main city of New Zealand, is designated the largest Polynesian city in the world.) There are also numbers of European immigrants from non-English-speaking origins, notably Holland and East Europe, and significant Indian (many from Fiji), Chinese and other South-East Asian groups.

Canada, whose population is about 30 million, is notable for its cultural diversity. The two main cultures are English-speaking and French-speaking European, and the indigenous people are the First Nations (formerly "Indians"), and the Inuit (formerly "Eskimos"). There are very large immigrant populations from European sources, the largest numbers being from the United Kingdom, Italy, Germany, Poland and Portugal. There are also substantial populations from India, Vietnam, the Caribbean, China and Hong Kong, with significant increases from Hong Kong in recent years as a result of its return to China in 1997.

Canada is officially a bilingual country, with 16% claiming that they were bilingual in 1991. In that year 15% reported that they were French speaking and 67% English speaking. Over the past decade or so, there has been a significant movement in Quebec toward the separation of that province from the rest of Canada, with a referendum in 1995 almost evenly split between those who favour Quebec separating and those favouring it remaining in Canada.

In addition to the bilingual nature of the country, there has been some support for multiculturalism in Canada from the federal government, although this appears to have weakened somewhat in recent years, perhaps due to the threatened separation of Quebec.

According to the 1991 census, there were approximately one million people in Canada with aboriginal origins at that time. This represents about 4% of the population. Of these, three-quarters were classified as Native Indians, 20% as Metis and 5% as Inuit. There has been somewhat of a revival of native culture in Canada in recent years, although perhaps not quite as strong as has been the case in New Zealand. As in New Zealand, land disputes are currently being worked on, although the process has been painfully slow. There is also a movement toward devolution of powers to native communities in Canada, which has been slow as well.

As far as PCHP is concerned, the experience of life, and the experience of power, health and well-being in that life, are determined to a large degree by "culture". The way we think, the way we relate to others, the priorities we have, the values, the patterns of living, the language—are all determined by what we might call "culture". Indeed, culture can be regarded as the broad patterns of living associated with different groupings in society, handed down from parents to their children, and moderated by the surrounding social and physical environment. While "ethnic" matters are often thought to be the only defining characteristic for the boundaries of a culture, clearly many groupings within broad ethnic populations have their own cultures or subcultures, which are also extremely important determinants of how people live, think, behave, feel and generally experience and operate in the world.

Culture is a subject that has conventionally been studied by anthropologists, who on the whole have tended to study "other cultures". Thus, culture is often, for many people, synonymous with, or closely linked to, ethnicity. One reason for culture being seen this way is our blindness to our own culture, whatever that might be. Our culture is seen as "normal" and "the way things are", whereas another culture is "different" and therefore "strange". Difficulties arise in most countries around culture, since there is almost inevitably one dominant group (which is not accustomed to thinking about or questioning its own "culture"), plus "other groups", whose "cultures" (ways of living) are different. Inevitably, because most people seem to have only a limited tolerance for cultural difference, and are often scared of it, the "lesser cultures" in whatever society they are, come under pressure to "change" and "adapt" to the dominant culture. That can be regarded, to put it charitably, as "human nature". Human nature or not, it is quite clear that being under pressure to change, or at least not being understood or appreciated in terms of one's own culture, is stressful for the people in those groupings. Not only does the stress itself threaten health, but often valuable practices for that people, used in the maintenance of life patterns and health, become dislocated or disappear, with consequent damaging effects on health. Simple justice, or even simple courtesy, would suggest that allowing people to retain their fundamental ways of living is the appropriate thing to do, and this is certainly the stance of PCHP. That is, we believe that each culture has its own intrinsic value, and should be honoured in those terms. At the same time, it is clear that all world cultures are under stress, as the "global village" becomes more and more accessible to international influences of commercialism and communication, so that all cultures are in constant flux and adaptation. Nevertheless, this change needs to be under the control of the people concerned as much as possible, rather than being forced deliberately, or being due to the ignorance of others. In short, cultural change and cultural behaviour are subject to the same laws of empowerment as the rest of PCHP. That is, we believe that any culture should be under the control of, and determined by, "the community" most affected, rather than being "dumped on" or forcibly made to change by others who think they "know best" or who ignore the sensibilities of others.

A good illustration in the health field of some of the points we are making here comes from a short book entitled *Talking Health but Doing Sickness: Studies in Samoan Health* by New Zealand anthropologist Patricia Kinloch (Kinloch, 1985). The Samoans being talked about here are from Western Samoa (to be distinguished from American Samoa), one of the largest South Pacific nations, with a population of 160 000. It is a very beautiful group of islands, with an energetic and proud people, and is perhaps best known throughout the West as the latter-day home of the novelist Robert Louis Stevenson. As mentioned, there are many Samoans in New Zealand (approximately 86 000), and Kinloch has studied Samoan culture in relation to health in both New Zealand and Western Samoa. Many health workers (including health promoters) of non-Samoan extraction work with Samoan people in New Zealand, and a lack of appreciation of how things are experienced from a Samoan perspective is often the result. Also, it is easy to jump to wrong conclusions about what is going on when cultural ways are viewed superficially. Kinloch says:

> Samoan culture, like any culture, comprises a totality of cultural practices, including healing practices, and is concerned with what it means to be human. People from various cultures have diverse ideas about what this means and they practise being human differently. Each group of people take their cultural ideas and practices for granted. (p. 13)

Kinloch then cites an earlier publication, written with fellow anthropologist Joan Metge (Metge and Kinloch, 1978), in which they define culture as a "system of shared understandings", certainly an experiential perspective.

> A culture can be simply and usefully defined as "a system of shared understandings"—understandings of what words and actions mean, of what things are really important, and of how these values should be expressed. These understandings are acquired in the process of growing up in a culture and most become so thoroughly internalised that we cease to be aware of them, coming to think of them (if at all) as "natural" or at least "second nature", not only the right but the only conceivable way of doing and looking at things, identifying "our way" as "the human way". (cited in Kinloch, 1985, p. 13)

She then goes on to note that it is when two cultures come in contact with each other that "culture" emerges as a conscious issue.

> So "natural" is our cultural commitment that it is only when we confront the understandings of another system that our words and actions can be seen to be different. The unthinking and unfeeling reaction to "otherness" is to regard the unknown culture as the one that is deviant or different; to make, in other words, an uninformed value judgement favouring one's self, one's own culture. (p. 13)

It is quite clear that different cultures *do* have fundamentally different ways of seeing the world, and acting in that world. And it is often quite an effort for someone from another culture to appreciate the complexities and subtleties of these differences. Even an intellectual understanding of a different concept often does not help much, if it is divorced from the cultural context and the "feel" of how someone in that culture thinks and experiences the world.

For example, Kinloch (a Westerner) is presumably mainly addressing a New Zealand *Papalagi* audience in the book we have been quoting (*Papalagi* is the Samoan equivalent of the Maori *Pakeha*, i.e. European) and the *Papalagi* health culture is a Western one. Even with the best will in the world, it is hard for such an audience to understand in a vacuum the fundamental differences between the way they see health, and the way a Samoan sees it. Here is how Kinloch talks about some of the basic differences in the views of disease and health:

> Sickness in the western view is an affair of the individual rather than an affair of the "people", where the word "people" signifies the series of relations which organise individuals into cultural, social, or family groups. Yet for the Samoan, "people" (*tagata*) signifies precisely that—a series of relations to other individuals, land and the world of the spirits, without which a being is not human, not a person. The health of a Samoan individual is so interwoven with the predicament of the social group as to be almost indistinguishable from it. (p. 15)

For most Westerners, it is possible to read this intellectually without having much sense of what is being said. Somewhat more of an idea can be got from an understanding of the Samoan social structure, and how the individual is tied to her or his extended family in ways that are usually not paralleled in Western society. Of the social structure, Kinloch says:

> Kinship is one of the most important metaphors underlying the organisation of social relations in Western Samoa. Most talk about social relations in Western Samoa is either about family relations of various extensions, or about the *matai* (chiefly) system. The kinship system and the *matai* system are interwoven. (p. 11)

In another book on Samoan life, *Faasamoa: The World of Samoans*, this time by a Samoan, Feletti Ngan-Woo (Ngan-Woo, 1990), the central role of extended family groups, called *aiga*, and the immersion of the individual in these groups, are clearly shown:

> Every Samoan has his or her roots in two extended families. These are the extended family of one's father and the extended family of one's mother. Each person has an important niche, a special place, and a special part to play within the *aiga* . . .
> Members of an *aiga* inherit an identity from birth. They are born into the support group of the *aiga*, and this *aiga* can be a very extended one. Family membership requires the allegiance of the individual to the *aiga*. Samoans, regardless of whether or not they live in an urban environment, in and out of Samoa, identify strongly with their *aiga* and they identify as strongly with their villages of origin. A number of *aiga* make up a village. A number of villages form a district. The totality of the districts constitute the country . . .
> Samoans expect their people to achieve, not for personal gain but in order to glorify God and for the good name of the *aiga* and the country. The *aiga* and *nuu* (village), therefore work towards this goal—the glorification of God. Similarly, the district and the nation call upon the people to work together for their district and for their country, with the ultimate aim of glorifying God. A person who is considered to be working for personal gain is sometimes described as *fia Papalagi*. The use of the term *fia Papalagi* has connotations of a dangerous generalisation concerning the *Pakeha*, for translated into English *fia Papalagi* means "wanting to be like a European". (pp. 9–10)

These short excerpts, then, show how the life of the Samoan individual is enmeshed in the *aiga*, and perhaps begins to show why the Samoan concept of illness and health is not the individualistic one of the European, but is more of a whole group phenomenon. It also shows how a lack of appreciation of the core values and structures of a culture can lead people outside that culture to be disempowering if they fail to take these things into account. These matters are not just "important" for Samoans; they are absolutely fundamental to their whole life. So, too, for people of any culture—there are fundamental matters that an outsider can fail to see, if an effort is not put into appreciating what that culture is about, and valuing whatever a culture might be.

An appreciation of another culture may strike at the very fundamentals of what *we* are about as health promoters. In the following passage from Kinloch, it is clear that a Western understanding of health and health promotion may be quite alien to Samoan ways of seeing the world.

> The Samoan notion of health is expressed in the words *soifua maloloina*. *Soifua* means "life", or "to live", and *maloloina* means "a rest", "health", or "to recover from sickness". Samoan people do not talk about health as if it were the absence of sickness, neither do they talk about sickness as if it were a fall from a state of complete well-being that is health. Health is not seen as something which can be promoted, neither is sickness seen as something which can be prevented or avoided. Samoan people do not seek better ways, in the sense of different or alternative methods, for preventing disease or disability.
>
> Samoan people see sickness as an inevitable, unpredictable and powerful discontinuity in the flow of life, a disruption of the social order. Westerners, on the other hand, usually do not accept disease as inevitable. Often they do not allow the body to heal itself. They want to intervene in the natural process of a disease and they expect a "cure" for everything. Despite the fact that Samoan people see sickness as inevitable, they also seek cares and cures. For them physical symptoms, a sick body, is not a sign of a "mechanical failure" but of the potential, and frequently real, sickness of the spirit. Spirit sickness is immanent in all Samoan sickness events. For Samoan people, "doing sickness" is seeking to re-establish the spiritual wholeness, not just of the sick person but also of the social group through the process of caring and curing the sick person. (pp. 15–16)

The point we are making here, then, is that cultures differ in the way they see the world, in their beliefs about health and sickness, and what they regard as important.

Now we want to move to another consideration, which relates in particular to the health and well-being of indigenous colonized people, that of the role of land, and the linkage of land to the three areas central to PCHP—quality of life, empowerment and community. In particular, we want to relate this analysis to the role of recognizing locality or place in health and health promotion.

COMMUNITY, LAND, POWER AND HEALTH: A MAORI PERSPECTIVE

The power of land in Maori culture and world view is shown in this passage written by Ranginui Walker, Professor of Maori Studies at the University of Auckland, and himself a Maori (Walker, 1982):

> The Maori people had been in occupation of the land they called Aotearoa [i.e. New Zealand] for a thousand years before systematic colonisation by Europeans began in 1840. From this prior occupation they derive status as *tangata whenua*

(people of the land). According to their mythology, Papatuanuku the Earth-mother and Ranginui the Sky-father were the first cause. They begat the gods who presided over the land, seas, forests, animals and plants.

From the bosom of the Earth-mother Tane the procreator fashioned Hineahu-one the Earth-formed-maid to establish the descent of man. Because man is derived from the Earth-mother who provides sustenance with food from her bosom, the earth was loved as a mother is loved.

At birth a child's *pito* (umbilical cord) was buried with accompanying rituals as an *iho-whenua* (connection with the land). For children of rank it was customary to plant a tree over the spot. Thereafter the tree was named for the child as his *iho-whenua*. It stood as an expression of man over the land and was cited in disputes over land boundaries.

Although the mythology of the Maori established the primacy of man over nature and validated his right to use the natural resources of the Earth-mother, myths, spiritual beliefs and customary usages indicated that man was not above nature. He was perceived as an integral part of nature and expected to relate to it in a responsible and meaningful way. (p. 69)

Today, the poor health statistics of Maori compared with *Pakeha* are attributed by Maori primarily to land issues. This is a concept that *Pakeha* can find hard to relate to. However, it becomes easier to understand when the integral relationship of the people with the land at a very deep and "spiritual" level is appreciated, and also when the history of colonization is understood.

In New Zealand at present, the symbol and rallying point of Maori cultural renaissance is the 1840 Treaty of Waitangi. Virtually every classroom in New Zealand has a copy of the Treaty on its walls, and all health meetings that involve Maori issues make primary reference to the Treaty. Basically, the Treaty of Waitangi is to do with land, and the "sovereignty" over—or in the empowerment language we use here, the "control over"—that land.

To make this point more strongly, to see some of the linkages between health, mental health, land and empowerment, and to learn more both about a cultural perspective and what this can contribute to PCHP, we wish to consider the Treaty of Waitangi further. Although it is a New Zealand issue, and one that continues to be near the top of the political, social and health agenda there, we trust the universals inherent in this discussion will become apparent.

The Treaty of Waitangi is a brief document. A literal translation of the Maori version is as follows:

This is the First. The Chiefs of the Confederation, and all those chiefs who have not joined in that Confederation, give up to the Queen of England for ever all the Governorship [*kawangatanga*] of their lands.

This is the Second. The Queen of England agrees and consents (to give) to the Chiefs, *hapus* [sub-tribes], and all the people of New Zealand the full

chieftainship [*rangatiratanga*] of their lands, their villages and all their posses-
sions [*taonga*, everything that is held precious] . . .

The focus in the Treaty is obviously land and its attendant resources. The
English and the Maori versions are slightly different, but certainly, by Maori
understanding, in return for giving up the overall nation to the British, they
were to retain sovereignty (*rangatiratanga*) over their tribal lands and posses-
sions. (The English version was that "the Chiefs and Tribes [were to have]
. . . the full and undisturbed possession of the Lands and Estates, Forests,
Fisheries, and other properties which they may collectively or individually
possess, so long as it is their wish and desire to maintain the same in their
possession . . .".)

Whichever version is used, the history of the following 150 years shows
that the Crown partners did not keep to their side of the bargain. Scores of
pieces of legislation passed during that time are evidence of a powerful
colonizing culture systematically taking land from the indigenous inhabitants by force or by legal device.

Early European accounts give a picture of Maori as a healthy, sophisticated, empowered people. The basis of this "cultural health" was land. In the
first few decades of European settlement, while Maori still had sovereignty
over and ownership of their land, they adapted very successfully to the new
reality, and flourished in that most Western of domains, namely commerce
and business (Williams, 1993). Had this continued, Maori today would undoubtedly still be in a state of high well-being, wealth and healthiness, as
they were then (apart from the ravages of Western diseases and vices, which
also took their toll). Today, as some of the basic land grievances are being
righted, and a new wealth and independence is coming into Maoridom,
some of the most successful major business developments in New Zealand
are under Maori control. However, the evidence is still there of the demoral-
ization and cultural destruction that took place as a result of the colonists'
efforts to wrest land from Maori, and to "disempower" them as a people.
For example, here are some data on Maori health and mental health in the
1990s (Bridgman, 1993; Patel, 1993):

First admission rates to psychiatric hospitals have fallen by up to 41% since
1970, except for Maori males where the admission rate has increased by 19%.

The suicide rate of Maori youth has increased sixfold over the last two decades.
Maori women have the highest rate of lung cancer of any group of women in
the world. It is 360% higher than the rate for non-Maori women . . . In the first
year of life, Maori children die at more than twice the rate of non-Maori . . .

[Overall] Maori rates of lung cancer are 240% greater than non-Maori; cervical
cancer is 320% higher; strokes are more than 200% higher; and motor vehicle
accidents are 150% higher.

Maori men are 47% of the men in the prison population and Maori women are 60% of the female population—equivalent to 1% of the total Maori population. [Maori are about 13% of the total New Zealand population.]

The central role of land in Maori life is clearly shown in another passage by Ranginui Walker (1982):

The *mana* [power, prestige] of a tribe was associated with a clearly defined territory. Boundaries were marked by physical features such as mountains, rivers, lakes, outcrops of rock or specially erected boundary markers. The integrity of the tribal territory was maintained by the ability of the group to hold and defend it against other tribes . . . An individual had rights to cultivation and a house site, but access to natural resources in tribal land was shared in common with other members of the tribe. (p. 70)

For Maori, then, health, well-being and a sense of community are closely linked to an aspect of community emphasized in PCHP, namely the locality. To Maori, community based on land and place is the most profound sort of community. To make this point more eloquently, we end this section with a quotation from the late John Rangihau (Rangihau, 1992), a noted leader of the Tuhoe people.

My sense of identity and commitment to Maori things is the result of history and traditions, and the fact that I grew up in a Maori community. In this community there was always a sense of the value of land and the emotional ties Maori have to it. As a result of these things I am strongly of the feeling that I am totally a New Zealander and cannot be regarded as anything else.

My education as a Maori was a matter of observation while I grew up in this complete community. It was a community where children were allowed to do their thing, where there was a place for the aged, and a place for the middle-aged. These places were within the structure of tribal organisation. I had to move through this as an apprenticeship for group living. We had to learn the dynamics of group living. We had to learn how to live together because we were in one another's pockets. If we didn't, problems would have arisen. From the time we were children we had to learn what it meant to be part of an extended family. We were warned not to do some things and we learned by others' experience.

The essence of community apprenticeship was young people learning by participating, by becoming carriers of wood, by chopping the wood and by setting up the *hangi* [oven in ground] . . . you progressed by observing and becoming involved in all the activities of the *marae* [sacred meeting place at the centre of community life]. That traditionally was the way a young man fitted into place as the elders died off.

Kinship bound us together in this situation. To me, kinship is the warmth of being together as a family group: what you can draw from being together and the strength of using all the resources of a family. And a strong feeling of *whanaua tanga* [kinship] reaches out to others in hospitality . . . I believe New Zealanders [generally] have been influenced by Maori hospitality laws. The whole basis of them is the business of showing concern for your neighbour, concern for him as a person, and therefore sharing his daily life and sharing the things of a community. And caring.

Whanaua tanga to me also means that whenever a person feels lonely he will go round and visit some of his kin and it is just as enjoyable for the kin to receive a visit as it is for the person to go. In other words there is as much joy— or perhaps greater joy—in giving as in receiving. And so we give of one another to one another—we give the talents we have so everybody can share in these sorts of experiences.

It may be a bit idealised but it has worked in our home areas over the years. It seems to me it could overcome some of the neuroses that urban dwellers are suffering because they are shut in. We should be harnessing our communities so they can become sharing, caring, and loving for *Pakeha* and Maori. But particularly for *Pakeha*: to overcome physical and mental breakdowns in the suburbs. I would hope to see the future planning of our cities and towns with more awareness of the need for people to socialise, to be able to come together as a group with common interests. Polynesian life should influence our whole thinking towards enjoying these sorts of things. (pp. 183–184)

A FIRST NATIONS PERSPECTIVE

Like the Maori, Canadian First Nations people have similar cultural and community strengths, which have also suffered because of the disruption of a colonizing culture and its land arrangements. The history of Canada is different, but underneath it is basically the same story, to which we now turn.

At the time of first European contact, Native peoples in what is now Canada existed as self-governing, independent nations or tribes that exercised control over geographic areas. Their authority was, however, eroded by the British and ultimately by the Canadian government when it accepted responsibility for discharging the provision of the treaties from the British under the British North American Act of 1867 and the Indian Act of 1876, which gave the Canadian minister responsible for Indian affairs complete control over Indians and their land (Little Bear et al., 1984). This control has been a focus of contention ever since.

One of the reasons why it has been contentious is that, in common with the Maori, Native peoples in Canada have placed extremely high value on their relationship with the land. The following statement, based on discussions with hundreds of Native people in the Canadian north, expresses it well:

We are telling you again and again that without the land Indian people have no soul, no life, no identity, no purpose. Control of the land is essential for our cultural and economic survival. (McCullum and McCullum, 1975)

On the other hand, it should be noted that the concept of nationhood and self-government among Canadian Native peoples is not exclusively geographically based. There are also cultural, philosophical, political, economic and social considerations. According to Leroy Little Bear and his colleagues, Native peoples "seek self-government so that they can develop their own institutions and shape laws to reflect and enhance their traditional cultural values". That is, "they want an Indian government that operates in accordance with traditional principles and customs, one that rests on a spiritual base and emphasizes group, not individual, rights" (Little Bear et al., 1984).

The latter point is especially important in that the concept of community in traditional Indian thought is expressed in "tribalism", as opposed to "individualism", which characterizes Western liberalism—for the Native, "involvement with his tribe was integral to his existence as a human being" (Little Bear et al., 1984).

Nevertheless, there is a very strong feeling among Native peoples in Canada that "land is the central issue" even though the concept of "private property" is in conflict with the Native value system (Little Bear et al., 1984). Thus, efforts by governments to disrupt the relationships between Natives and the land have resulted in significant consequences for Native communities, leading, to some extent at least, to the collapse of their traditional "healthy" cultures, which were based on a "natural" and "spiritual" relationship between peoples and their land. This disruption may have contributed to many of the problems faced by Native communities in Canada, which are not too dissimilar from the problems noted in the case of the Maori. That is, Natives in Canada have had, and continue to experience, higher death rates, lower life expectancy, higher rates of alcohol problems, higher rates of smoking, and higher rates of incarceration than their counterparts in the general population.

It is our view that the cultural values that have to do with the relationship of people to the land have at the very least to be acknowledged and respected. Moreover, it is our feeling that through a PCHP approach to community, it may be possible to build on these values and make them the foundation for healthy communities and lives.

CONCLUSION

In this chapter we have introduced the concept of culture to the health promotion discourse or, at least, to the version of it represented by PCHP. It is obviously not possible to do justice to such a topic in the space available here. What we have tried to do is show that culture is close to how it was characterized by Metge and Kinloch (1978)—a system of shared understandings we hold in common with those other people who constitute "our culture". These understandings are so "thoroughly internalized" that we are barely aware of them, yet they are the basis of the whole way we see, experience and interact with the world. A failure to grasp this by health promoters is likely to be extremely disempowering to those we work with. That is, "personal power" comes from a sense of efficacy, strength, belonging in the world, and the esteem in which we are held by others. The extent to which another person or group tries to get us to see or do things in another way is not only an insult, but will strike at the heart of our being in a way that will jeopardize our health and mental health. Furthermore, our very concept of the nature of health and mental health, and what are their determinants, will be intimately tied up with our "culture". At the very least, health promoters operating from a PCHP perspective need to "honour" culture. But better, they need to work in a way that strengthens culture, and the sense of identity and strength that everyone derives from their culture.

Probably those cultures most under threat in the modern world are indigenous cultures who have been colonized. For them, the issue of land is an especially acute one. The examples we have given here of the role of land in Maori and First Nations culture (and health) are testimony to this. These examples, from a PCHP perspective, are important from another point of view as well. They remind many of us from dominant, Western style cultures of something we may have forgotten—of the importance of land, sense of place and community for health and well-being generally. If community development is to be an important part of the health promotion enterprise, then the role of land, place and locality will need to have increased attention.

Certainly these matters touch deep parts of our being, and have an important role to play in any consideration of promoting health, mental health and quality of life on an enduring basis.

8

SPIRITUAL DIMENSIONS

If culture is a topic that lies at the periphery of most contemporary health promotion considerations, then spirituality is even more so. Yet, like culture, spirituality may be considered a core concern of health promotion. Certainly, numerous health promotion workers, as well as many "ordinary community people", have strong interests in this area, but there is not yet the language, the professional permission, or the academic base to put this subject "out there" in the public domain.

This chapter is a preliminary attempt to put spirituality (as distinct from religion) on the health promotion agenda. To some extent we feel we are "flying blind" in uncharted territory. Also, we (the two authors) differ considerably in our thoughts and feelings about this area and its relevance to health promotion. It is important to acknowledge that, because this area involves a level of abstraction, a depth of subjectivity and an inadequate language for its communication, its existence in a conventional "academic" setting is difficult. Notwithstanding, spirituality, or the "transpersonal", is a fundamental dimension for PCHP.

THE MEANING OF "TRANSPERSONAL"

In academic psychology, the term "spiritual" is replaced by the term "transpersonal". Although the two terms are not exactly synonymous, the term "transpersonal", while clumsy linguistically, captures a dimension that makes it relevant to the preoccupations of PCHP. That is, translated literally, it means "beyond the personal", which relates it directly to the power of the collective, as in community or culture, and to the putting of "other" before "self".

According to psychiatrist Roger Walsh and psychologist Frances Vaughan, editors of *Paths Beyond Ego: The Transpersonal Vision* (Walsh and Vaughan, 1993), at the heart of transpersonal considerations are "transpersonal experiences". This resonates well with our approach here, which is first and foremost an experiential one. In the introductory chapter to their book, they say:

Transpersonal experiences may be defined as experiences in which the sense of identity or self extends beyond (trans) the individual or personal to encompass aspects of humankind, life, psyche and cosmos formerly experienced as other. (p. 3)

These transpersonal experiences are studied by a number of disciplines, including psychology, psychiatry, sociology, anthropology, ecology, religious studies and philosophy. The area is not necessarily to do with "religion", a belief in God or any other especially "spiritual" concept, although it can include these:

The transpersonal disciplines or their practitioners [are not associated with] any specific interpretation of transpersonal experience. In particular they do not tie the disciplines to any particular ontology, metaphysics or worldview, nor to any specific doctrine, philosophy or religion . . . Transpersonal experiences have long been interpreted in many different ways and this will doubtless continue. A transpersonalist could be religious or nonreligious, theist or atheist, Taoist or Jewish. (p. 4)

Walsh and Vaughan say that there are a number of themes that keep recurring in definitions of the transpersonal area, and it is worth considering these briefly to make a little more sense of what is involved here. They outline six of these in transpersonal psychology, to do with the nature of the transpersonal ontology, the "self", ultimate values, highest potentials, states of consciousness, and health. At least three of these—the "self", highest potentials and health—are relevant to our present discussion.

Ontological assumptions include the presupposition that "a transcendent reality underlies and binds together all phenomena" . . .
    Several definitions refer to a transcendent "Self" while others indicate that transpersonal psychology represents a contemporary exploration of the perennial philosophy [which talks of an "eternal Self"] . . .
    Several definitions refer to ultimates, suggesting that transpersonal psychology's primary concern is with ultimate dimensions of human experience . . . and "humanity's highest potential" . . .
    Many definitions define transpersonal psychology in terms of the study of altered states of consciousness . . .
    Other definitions assume the field is centrally concerned with psychological health and wellbeing . . . Our own definition in *Beyond Ego* [the earlier edition of *Paths Beyond Ego*] said that the field was "concerned with the study of psychological health and wellbeing". (unpublished manuscript)

For our purposes, the discussion on culture in Chapter 7 provides a good context for the way we wish to approach the transpersonal area. As can be seen from the Walsh and Vaughan outline, the "transpersonal" has to do with the "highest", "ultimate", "healthiest" and "transcendent" aspects of life, and hence is relevant to PCHP, which is also about such matters. Also, it is quintessentially an *experiential* area of study, which may be one reason it does not get much attention from conventional science. Both cultural and transpersonal issues may best be seen in terms of their subjective or experiential aspects, as senior Anglican clergyman and former navy chaplain Maori Marsden (his first name is "Maori", as well as his being Maori in his ethnicity) says in a chapter called "God, man and universe: A Maori view" (Marsden, 1992):

> The route to *Maoritanga* [Maori culture] through abstract interpretation is a dead way. The way can only lie through a passionate subjective approach. That is more likely to lead to a goal.
> As a person brought up within the culture, who has absorbed the values and attitudes of the Maori, my approach to Maori things is largely subjective. The charge of lacking objectivity does not concern me: the so-called objectivity some insist on is simply a form of arid abstraction, a model or a map. It is not the same thing as the taste of reality . . . (p. 117)

> Only an approach which sets out to explore and describe the main features of the consciousness in the experience of the Maori offers any hope of adequate coverage. For the reality we experience subjectively is incapable of rational synthesis. This is why so many Maori react against the seemingly facile approach of foreign anthropologists to the attitudes, mores and values, and the affective states of mind which produce them . . .
> Remembering that the cultural milieu is rooted both in the temporal world and the transcendent world, this brings a person into intimate relationship with the gods and his universe. (pp. 136–137)

The term "transpersonal", then, relates to those aspects of human experience where the ordinary, limited, self-centred self is somehow put to one side, and a "greater picture" or "higher picture" is revealed. Subjectively, this experience, or rather set of experiences, has been well documented. Sometimes it is alluded to as "mystical", but this is a misleading term. Some such experiences may be "mystical", in that the sense of going beyond or outside the normal confines of the ordinary self has a "numinous" quality about it—that is, the person feels strongly that he or she has been in contact with a "higher", "transcendent" or "vaster" power or presence of some sort, to which a name like "God" might be given. But it is clear that this is only one kind of transpersonal experience. There are many others too, including what we are most concerned with here—a sense of connectedness with others, with the environment, with things as they are in the everyday world. Although this sounds quite ordinary, and in a way it is, at the same time we feel that the experience is somehow "deep", "important", and very fundamental and meaningful in a significant way, which may be difficult to express in words, but which "feels right". Many people who work in community projects express this sense in a variety of ways. This experience is usually accompanied by certain emotional experiences or "tones"—of liberation, profundity, joy, wonder, "doing something important and worthwhile", and so on. Sometimes the experiences are sudden, intense and brief. At other times they are more or less permanent, giving a sense of a life transformed in a significant way. In almost all cases, they leave a profound impression. Furthermore, transpersonal experiences may be quite common. For example, if "altered states of consciousness" are taken as a defining dimension of the transpersonal, these appear to figure in almost all cultures:

> Of a sample of 488 societies, in all parts of the world, for which we have analyzed the relevant ethnographic literature, 437 or 90% are reported to have one or more institutionalized, culturally patterned, forms of altered states of consciousness. This . . . suggests that we are, indeed, dealing with a matter of major importance, not merely a bit of anthropological esoteric. It is clear that we are dealing with a psychological capacity available to all societies, and that, indeed, the vast majority of societies have used it in their own particular ways . . . (Bourguignon, 1973, p. 11)

Certainly, the experiences vary greatly, and we cannot hope to do justice to them here. We just know that they are usually interpreted as the most important things that ever happen to people, and that somehow they represent "spiritual health" or "ultimate sanity". Here are a few reported examples of how people express transpersonal experiences:

> Am totally at peace at peace . . .
> Am supremely free free free free free.
> Should I be so happy?
> (A Japanese businessman, following a Zen experience. Quoted by Kapleau, 1965, p. 207)

> I felt a great inexplicable joy, a joy so powerful that I could not restrain it, but had to break into song, a mighty song, with room for the one word: joy, joy! . . . And then in the midst of such a fit of mysterious and overwhelming delight I became a shaman, not knowing myself how it came about. But I was a shaman. I could see and hear in a totally different way. I had gained my . . . enlightenment. (An Eskimo, quoted by Neher, 1980, p. 106)

> Towards the end of the 1950's, the various negative aspects of my life had made me into a neurotic, incapable of being loving, inhibited, apprehensive and with a gloomy cast of mind which sometimes impelled me to long for death as the only way out of an unendurable existence . . .
> [Later, after the death of a close friend, I was suddenly filled with] a "knowing" more vivid and real than anything I have ever experienced in the literal sense. It was as if for a moment one had known reality and in comparison the world of the senses was the dream. I was filled with an unutterable joy, which I shall never be able to describe . . . From the day of what I can only consider my rebirth, my neurotic difficulties disappeared and have never since returned. (An English woman, quoted by Cohen and Phipps, 1979, pp. 78–79)

Just in case anyone reading this should feel that he or she does not know what we are talking about here, William James, whose classic book *The Varieties of Religious Experience* (James, 1902) represents an early example of an experiential approach in academic psychology, said this about a very common Western "transpersonal experience":

> The sway of alcohol over mankind is unquestionably due to its power to stimulate the mystical faculties of human nature, usually crushed to earth by the cold facts and dry criticisms of the sober hour. Sobriety diminishes, discriminates, and says no; drunkenness expands, unites, and says yes. It is in fact the great exciter of the *Yes* function in man. It brings its votary from the chill periphery of things to the radiant core. It makes him for the moment one with truth. (pp. 304–305)

In short, then, the transpersonal experience or, rather, set of experiences are reasonably universal, and are the "supreme" or most highly valued experiences in all or most cultures. They have a variety of qualities about them relevant to us here—of power, health, mental health, love or goodwill to others, community-building, a lowering of negative emotions, a diminution of self-centredness, joy, liberation, certainty, tranquillity, equanimity and a variety of other positive, "healthy", socially constructive dimensions relevant to the goals of PCHP. Most important, these experiences seem to bring people in touch with what can be regarded as the ultimate in their existence, the ultimate "quality of life".

A proper study of these matters would require a whole book in itself. Here, we would like to limit ourselves to the immediate themes of this book—empowerment, community, and the growth of health and quality of life. But before we do this, we would like to set the discussion in the context of the overall area, for which we use the term "Perennial Philosophy", coined by Leibnitz in the 18th century, and popularized by Aldous Huxley in a book of that name (Huxley, 1961).

THE PERENNIAL PHILOSOPHY

Because the spiritual area is hard to grasp, takes so many forms, and involves the most profound dimensions and interpretations of both how we see ourselves as people and how we see the universe we inhabit, it is little wonder that there are so many versions of it. Every culture appears to have its religion, spiritual life, "states of consciousness", magic, ethical system, shamanship, psychology and so on, and these all impinge on the area of transpersonal experience. In the realm of religion alone, it is clear that not only are there enormous differences in systems of belief around the world, and in concepts of God or His/Her/Its equivalent, but also people are passionately attached to their religious systems, as is evident from the religious warfare and sectarianism that is a feature both of past and present world events. So to take a "neutral" yet involved stance here is difficult. Of all the options, we believe the overall view provided by Huxley's analysis of the "Perennial Philosophy" is the most helpful, even though it has had its critics (see Walsh and Vaughan, 1993), and is also expressed in the culturally and gender insensitive language one might expect of an Englishman in the 1940s.

According to Huxley (1962), the Philosophia Perennis (Leibnitz' term) is the "Highest Common Factor" in "the traditionary lore of primitive peoples in every region of the world, and in its fully developed forms it has a place in every one of the higher religions".

> In Vedanta and Hebrew prophecy, in the Tao The King [*Tao Te Ching*] and the Platonic dialogues, in the Gospel according to St John and Mahayana [Buddhist] theology, in Plotinus and the Areopagite, among the Persian Sufis and the Christian mystics of the Middle Ages and the Renaissance—the Perennial Philosophy has spoken almost all the languages of Asia and Europe and has made use of the terminology and traditions of every one of the higher religions. But under all this confusion of tongues and myths, of local histories and particularist doctrines, there remains a Highest Common Factor, which is the Perennial Philosophy in what might be called its chemically pure state . . . [However], it is only in the act of contemplation, when words and even personality are transcended, that the pure state of the Perennial Philosophy can actually be known. The records left by those who have known it in this way make it abundantly clear that all of them, whether Hindu, Buddhist, Hebrew, Taoist, Christian or Mohammedan, were attempting to describe the same essentially indescribable Fact. (1962, pp. 11–12)

The difficulty of putting the essence of the Perennial Philosophy into words is widely acknowledged. For example, the famous opening lines of the *Tao Te Ching*, reputedly the most widely read spiritual document in history, are as follows:

> The Tao that can be told is not the eternal Tao.
> The name that can be named is not the eternal name.
> The nameless is the beginning of heaven and earth.
> (Feng and English, 1972, p. 2)

Notwithstanding this inexpressibility, Huxley tells us it is possible to delineate "four fundamental doctrines" which lie at the core of the Perennial Philosophy:

> First: the phenomenal world of matter and of individualized consciousness— the world of things and animals and men and even gods—is the manifestation of a Divine Ground within which all partial realities have their being, and apart from which they would be nonexistent.

Second: human beings are capable not merely of knowing *about* the Divine Ground by inference; they can also realize its existence by a direct intuition, superior to discursive reasoning. This immediate knowledge unites the knower with that which is known.

Third: man possesses a double nature, a phenomenal ego and an eternal Self, which is the inner man, the spirit, the spark of divinity within the soul. It is possible for a man, if he so desires, to identify himself with the spirit and therefore with the Divine Ground, which is of the same or like nature with the spirit.

Fourth: man's life on earth has only one end and purpose: to identify himself with his eternal Self and so to come to unitive knowledge of the Divine Ground. (1962, p. 13)

In the context of PCHP, two of these principles are especially relevant, namely the third and fourth. The fourth implies that until we come to a realization of our "true nature", to use the Buddhist term, we will not have fulfilled what we are here for, and will therefore remain in a fundamental state of discontent or "unwellness". And there is no doubt that most "spiritual searches" are fuelled by a sense of existential discontent with the way things are, or the way one is.

The third principle, that of a "phenomenal ego" and an "eternal Self", is perhaps the most crucial for us here, although this dichotomy may be a bit misleading. That is, there is not necessarily just one monolithic, ultimate Reality beyond the "phenomenal ego", but perhaps many layers. For example, many cultures see "community" as a wider reality beyond the immediate self-preoccupations of the individual, and naturally we would support this view. In the earlier cited book by Feleti Ngan-Woo on Samoan life (Ngan-Woo, 1990), we read that:

> The social structure of Samoan society is held together and is actively maintained, by an adherence to unwritten but universally understood cultural conventions. These conventions govern the formalised giving and receiving of *ava* (respect), of *faaloalo* (reverence), and *alofa* (love, compassion and concern). These three practices are the basis of spiritual and cultural living. Respect, reverence and love are seen as qualities acceptable to God and hence necessary in the practice of *faaSamoa*. (p. 9)

In short, the aspects of the transpersonal we are most interested in here are where the "phenomenal ego", the self-centred self of the individual, is softened in the interests of a larger and more "profound" purpose, which is somehow connected with some ultimate reality. (Whether or not one wants to use a term like "divine", as Huxley does, is a matter of personal preference. It is not a term we will use here. On the other hand, the failure to use such a term should not blind us to the fact that we are referring to levels of reality beyond normal words, and which are real, legitimate, mysterious and profound.)

Having set the foundation for this discussion, we can now go on to look in a little more detail at some key concepts of PCHP from this perspective.

POWER AND THE TRANSPERSONAL

Some of the persistent themes that come through in the transpersonal area are concepts to do with energy and power. For example, there have been a number of attempts in recent years (e.g. Capra, 1987; Goswami, 1993; Zukav, 1979) to link modern quantum physics with transpersonal experience, on the premise that the "Divine Ground" as Huxley calls it, that is, the ultimate reality behind the world as we see it with our senses, is close to what physics has been uncovering for the past century.

Modern physics has been revolutionized by the approach called "quantum mechanics", and it is this approach which has given us many of the marvels of the modern, technological world—the transistor, the computer, the semi-conductor, and so on. It has also given us nuclear weapons. The term "quantum" itself was first used in 1900 by the German Max Planck, to describe the way in which electrons emitted or absorbed energy in discrete amounts, which he called "quanta" (see Goswami, 1993). This was followed by Einstein, who in 1905 "suggested that light exists as a quantum, a discrete bundle of energy—that we now call a photon", and Bohr, who in 1913 "applied the idea of light quanta to suggest that the whole world of the atom is full of quantum jumps" (see Goswami, 1993). And it is, of course, the atom that underlies the whole of what we see and sense as the material world. In short, then, quantum physics tells us that, at least at one level, the whole of reality can be seen as an organized energy system, rather than as "solid" matter. An atom is mainly "space", the components of which are high-density energy, and which are held in relation to each other by energy. So energy, for which one can also read "power", is reasonably fundamental in the scheme of things.

What is also interesting here is how it becomes necessary to conceptualize reality in terms of its interconnectedness, especially in terms of its "group behaviour", rather than just seeing it in terms of discrete events or units, which is the custom in conventional reductionist science.

> Quantum mechanics concerns itself only with group behaviour. It intentionally leaves vague the relation between group behaviour and individual events because individual subatomic events cannot be determined accurately (the uncertainty principle) and, as we shall see in high-energy particles, they constantly are changing. Quantum physics abandons the laws which govern individual events and states *directly* the statistical laws which govern collections of events. Quantum mechanics can tell us how a group of particles will behave, but the only thing it can say about an individual particle is how it *probably* will

behave. Probability is the major characteristic of quantum mechanics. (Zukav, 1979, p. 60)

Here, we do not want to make a too facile jump between the laws and procedures of atomic and subatomic physics and the social world of people and the community. However, we constantly read in the transpersonal traditions, especially those of the East, some sort of imagery like "the universe is contained in a grain of sand", which leads us to suppose that what is deemed (by those traditions) to happen at the "micro" level is also true at the "macro" level. But even as a convenient metaphor, we see that at the very heart of the nature of things are the concepts of energy, power relations, interconnectedness and "group behaviour", and while the "individual" still counts, he, she or it figures less prominently than in other analyses of reality. Also, there is deemed to be a vast underlying order, or "ground of being", which is the context for all levels of activity, subatomic or human.

COMMUNITY AND THE TRANSPERSONAL SELF

In an earlier part of this chapter, we made reference to the role of the self from a community perspective, where the interests of the total community or social setting can render less potent the preoccupations of the self-centred self. This is accompanied by a valued sense of being part of a larger reality or "self", and this experience of being part of what is usually regarded as outside oneself is what really defines the concept of transpersonal. Here, we want to make the case that the wish to be part of a larger reality that is community is deeply embedded in us as human beings, and probably comes from our atavistic history as members of tribes and social groupings on which our whole survival and life depended. In short, we would share the view with the community psychologist, Seymour B. Sarason, that there is an "overarching" value or wish in human beings for a "psychological sense of community", which may be pushed to one side in the face of the realities of modern living styles, but is nevertheless there (Sarason, 1974).

From a transpersonal perspective, this wish to be part of a larger community can be seen as having to do with the concept of "self". (The concepts of self and ego seem to have been central to the Perennial Philosophy in its various forms in virtually every culture and age.) According to most transpersonal traditions, the major cause of human suffering, violence, discontent, exploitation and social breakdown is to do with the assertion of the "phenomenal ego". According to most traditions, while this ego or self is what causes most personal and social harm, it is actually a falsehood, an illusion. So the question is: What is this self?

In the book *Beyond Therapy*, its editor, the English psychologist and Buddhist Guy Claxton, contributes a chapter called "The light's on but there's nobody home: The psychology of no-self" (Claxton, 1986). In this he says:

> The central assertion of Buddhism is that we are all living our lives on the basis of mistakes, and that, because we have not spotted these mistakes, we create for ourselves unnecessary suffering . . .
>
> One of these conceptual mistakes—or rather one cluster of them—is seen as being crucial, for it functions as the lynch-pin that keeps all the others locked in place . . . Through constant training in early childhood, all the more effective for being implicit . . . we acquire an unnecessary view of ourselves. Mostly we are unaware of holding this view, or *any* view, at all, and to the extent that we do notice it, it seems natural and inevitable. But if our "sense of self" is *second* nature to us, we might wonder what was the *first*: what Zen calls our "original face"?
>
> The sense of self is hard to examine because it forms the stage on which all our actions are performed, the screen onto which all our experience is projected; and if it is untrue, warped or slanted, then the whole drama of a life is distorted . . . But those who pursue [a] critical [self-]examination to the end are, like "those who go down to the woods today", sure of a Big Surprise—there is no stage, no screen, no ground, no experience, no knower, no self. It is all going on in mid-air. (p. 52)

According to Claxton, the false sense of self has three characteristics—that of separateness, of persistence, and of autonomy. That is, we feel that "I" am on my own in this life, and "I" need to keep a grip on things over time, so that "I", on which my whole fate and survival depends, can stay in control. The corollary of this is that if we "trust" our environment, trust others around us, and trust the flow of life generally, we can relax our dependence on this phony "I", and "flow" with life in an easy way. This is the "liberation" we spoke of earlier. But, instead, we go on acting as though "I" have to control everything. As Claxton says:

> This sense of a Self that is the cause, and therefore in control, of at least some of what I think and do is crucial. I reason, I decide, I intend, I evaluate, and sometimes I change my mind. Behind the act is an actor whose initiative entitles him to any praise or blame that accrues. I am, and feel, responsible. (p. 55)

We suggest that "losing" oneself in community action and sense of community is one avenue to weakening the role of this self (as is, indeed, losing oneself in any activity where one is taken "outside" oneself to a "greater" cause). Claxton reflects this in saying that as he loses his ego-self, he becomes a "better neighbour":

> As I relax into myself I get more and more in touch with my unity, the wholeness and integrity that my *theory* [about the nature of my self] has denied. And

much of the uneasiness and tension in my life, that my theory had told me was inevitable and even valuable, begins to disappear. Guilt, shame, embarrassment, self-doubt, self-consciousness, fear of failure and much anxiety ebb away, and as I do so I seem to become, contrary to expectations, a better neighbour. As I can look inwards with more acceptance and compassion, so I can look outwards at others. My needs to dominate and censure, to be wary and manipulative, they melt too. It is truly startling to discover how much of the mischief and misery in the world is attributable to this simple ontological mistake. (p. 69)

THE SPIRITUAL IN SOCIAL AND COMMUNITY ACTION

Today, there are many people working in the helping and social professions and agencies who have a central interest in spiritual matters, ranging from the work being done by "liberation theology" priests in South America, through the Hindu projects initiated at the village level by Mahatma Gandhi in India, to Deep Ecology in America, and to Buddhist projects such as the Sarvodaya Shramadana movement in Sri Lanka (Ariyaratne, 1985). Here we just want to draw attention to this area, and look at one or two aspects relevant to PCHP. The emphasis we want to make is that of the Perennial Philosophy, so that the concept of transpersonal self remains the dominant theme. This being the case, our emphasis is more on the Eastern approach, which takes this as a central part of their world view, than on the more conventional Christian or Judaic approach.

Here, our starting point is the 1976 book by British social worker David Brandon, called *Zen in the Art of Helping*. Brandon's particular interest is homelessness, and he was director of a government-sponsored research project on homeless young people.

According to Brandon:

> An important aspect of genuine caring lies in the continuing capacity to put one's self-interest second to that of the client's needs. We are striving for *his* greater independence rather than enhancing our personal feelings of power . . . [At the same time] helping is not socialized masochism and the helper has also a right to satisfaction, joy and love from the process. (p. 27)

Brandon then goes on to quote his Zen teacher, Irmgard Schloegl, in her book *The Wisdom of the Zen Masters* (Schloegl, 1975). This illustrates well the way our own self-preoccupied way of looking at things through our ego can often cause damage, whereas seeing with the non-ego self does the opposite.

> [Through the non-ego self, there arises] the virtue of seeing clearly and of being able to act in accordance with that seeing. This embraces all the truly human

qualities, such as responsibility, justice, consideration, warmth of heart, joy, tolerance, compassion, awareness of strength of personality and its power and limits.
For nobody has the right to manipulate anybody or to impress anybody with his
stronger personality, not even for the other's imagined good, for nobody can
know what that good is. This is courtesy rather than callousness, for the other's
dignity is thus acknowledged, or the dignity of his grief is respected. If and when
he is ready, the other will of himself reach out for consolation and feel free to ask
for a hand to point out the way. (Schloegl, 1975, p. 12)

Central to understanding the non-ego self approach to helping others is
the concept of compassion. This, and its close relative "love", is recognized
by most or all transpersonal traditions as being one of the hallmarks of a
transpersonal approach.

Compassion is an unpopular word these nowadays. It points toward commitment, involvement, caring, love and generosity of heart. These are directions
closely related to feeling and sentiment, sources of considerable embarrassment for twentieth-century man. It is less dangerous to be cool than passionate
in contemporary society . . .
    Openness, intimacy and sensitivity are the herbs of compassion. Those
qualities are concerned with seeing deeply and directly into the other person and
feeling his needs and wants. That has nothing to do with verbal diarrhoea. Being
compassionate does not mean giving people the everlasting benefit of your
advice . . . Genuine caring is much less conspicuous and unselfconscious . . .
    Compassion is the process of deep contact with the primordial source of
love. It is the direct communication from the innermost recesses of one's
existence.
    When a person develops real compassion, he is uncertain whether he is
being generous to others or to himself because compassion is environmental
generosity, without direction, without "for me" and without "for them". It is
filled with joy, spontaneously existing joy, constant joy in the sense of trust, in
the sense that joy contains tremendous wealth, richness. (Tibetan Buddhist
teacher Chogyam Trungpa, 1973, p. 99)

Brandon (1976) introduces us to the concept of "Taoistic change". This
principle sums up what we are aiming for in PCHP "intervention".
    In Taoism, an ancient Chinese spiritual tradition, the Tao is regarded as
"the flow of nature", the organic way things are, the energy system behind
all reality. According to Alan Watts, in his book *Tao: The Watercourse Way*
(Watts, 1975), the Tao has the characteristics of flowing water:

Thus the Tao is the course, the flow, the drift, or the process of nature, and I call
it the Watercourse Way because both Lao-Tzu and Chuang-Tzu [who, in the
5th century BC, wrote the two classic works of Taoism] use the flow of water as
its principal metaphor . . . (p. 44)

The principle for health promotion work is that we "intervene" as little as
possible, and certainly not in a sudden, "quick fix", or "blitz" way. Rather,

the work we do is "organic", gently assisting with the processes that are already there, but which may require nurturing to bring to fruition.

> The principle is that if everything is allowed to go its own way the harmony of the universe will be established, since every process in the world can "do its own thing" in relation to all others. The political analogy is Kropotkin's anarchism—the theory that if people are left alone to do as they please, to follow their nature and discover what truly pleases them, a social order will emerge of itself. Individuality is inseparable from community. (Watts, 1975, p. 43)

These considerations in turn have something to say about how to work in a PCHP way. For example, Brandon quotes Abraham Maslow's defining of a Taoistic approach, which comes close to our approach in PCHP:

> [Taoistic means] self-regulation, self-government and the self-choice of the organism . . . Taoistic means asking rather than telling. It means non-intruding, non-controlling. It stresses non-interfering observation rather than controlling manipulation. It is receptive and passive rather than active and forceful. (Maslow, 1973, p. 15)

Brandon adds:

> It assumes that the other side has a reasonable point of view—a slice of the truth. It is opposed to people management and has no hard and delineated aims in its relations to people. It is optimistic about the nature of human beings. It holds that the organism naturally searches for both physical and mental health. (p. 88)

At the same time, to work in this non-controlling, non-manipulative way is difficult for most of us.

> It is very hard to flow [in the way we are talking about here]. It becomes harder still to give up those ambitions for the control and changing of others; the simple desire to appear important, to have, to be popular and lovable . . .
> I feel this powerful urge to tell people what to do. There is a great drive deep inside to manage people's lives, that only I know what really ought to happen. Hard-shelled ego. Often I would rather pretend that controlling desire is not there at all. It mainly feeds and enlarges my own pot-bellied ego. (pp. 90–91)

Brandon then makes what is perhaps the most radical statement of all:

> Not to intervene at all can be the best form of action. Research into the results of intervening through group-work, psychotherapy and even community development programmes, makes very depressing reading. We need to review not only the end result but also the motivating energy. Why did we seek to intervene at all? Was it a simple expression of our feelings that we were right and the desire to "have our own way"? (p. 93)

Brandon quotes Charles Reich, who, like Maori Marsden (see earlier in this chapter), argues for the value of a "radical subjectivity". According to Reich:

> To start from self does not mean to be selfish. It means to start from premises based on human life and the rest of nature, rather than premises that are the artificial products of the Corporate State, such as power and status. It is not an "ego trip" but a radical subjectivity designed to find genuine values in a world whose official values are false and distorted. It is not egocentricity, but honesty, wholeness, genuineness in all things. It starts from self because human life is found as individual units, not as corporations and institutions; its intent is to start from life. (quoted by Brandon, 1976, pp. 94–95)

The best we can do, it seems, is to "know ourselves"—to recognize, as does Brandon, the inclinations in each of us for power and control over others, to be superior, important and loved, while also recognizing that we probably have something of benefit and importance to bring to the people and communities with whom it is our wish to work. The optimal approach, we would suggest, to any situation in which we might want to work, is one of caution—listening, being aware, knowing our own ego-driven pro-clivities, flowing with what is there, knowing that the situation has its own solutions potentially in it, believing in the people, and gently nurturing and supporting the strengths that are there. We cannot do nothing, and no one is asking us to. But the next best option is to proceed in the compassionate, Taoistic way.

We give the last word here to Thich Nhat Hanh, a Vietnamese Buddhist teacher now resident in France, nominated by Martin Luther King for the Nobel Peace Prize for his work during the Vietnam War, and who now works with refugees from South-East Asia. In his book *Being Peace* (Nhat Hanh, 1987), he says that what counts is not our external work for peace or for a better world, but the "state of being" we bring to it.

> Many of us worry about the situation of the world. We don't know when the bombs will explode. We feel that we are on the edge of time. As individuals, we feel helpless, despairing. The situation is so dangerous, injustice is so wide-spread, the danger is so close. In this kind of situation, if we panic, things will only become worse. We need to remain calm, to see clearly . . .
>
> I like to use the example of a small boat crossing the Gulf of Siam. In Vietnam, there are many people, called boat people, who leave the country in small boats. Often the boats are caught in rough seas or storms, the people may panic, and boats can sink. But even if one person aboard can remain calm, lucid, knowing what to do and what not to do, he or she can help the boat survive. His or her expression—face, voice—communicates clarity and calm-ness, and people have trust in that person. They will listen to what he or she says. One such person can save the lives of many.
>
> Our world is something like a small boat. Compared with the cosmos, our planet is a very small boat. We are about to panic because our situation is no better than the situation of the small boat in the sea. You know that we have

more than 50,000 nuclear weapons. Human kind has become a very dangerous species. We need people who can sit still and be able to smile, who can walk peacefully . . .

Children understand very well that in each woman, in each man, there is a capacity of waking up, of understanding, and of loving. Many children have told me that they cannot show me anyone who does not have this capacity. Some people allow it to develop, and some do not, but everyone has it. This capacity of waking up, of being aware of what is going on in your feelings, in your body, in your perceptions, in the world, is called Buddha nature, the capacity of understanding and loving. Since the baby of that Buddha is in us, we should give him or her a chance. Smiling is very important. If we are not able to smile, then the world will not have peace. It is not by going out for a demonstration against nuclear missiles that we can bring about peace. It is with our capacity of smiling, breathing, and being peace that we can make peace. (pp. 9, 11)

III

THE PRACTICE OF PCHP

In Part III, we take the principles that have been outlined so far, and look at how they can be applied in practice. This is done through the vehicle of a procedural approach called the People System. We start, in Chapter 9, by considering general issues. Then in Chapter 10, we introduce the People System in more detail, showing how to use it. In Chapter 11 we look at the issue of how to do outcome evaluation within a People System framework. Then in Chapters 12–14, we look at the actual application of this system to a series of real-life projects. Although fairly precise procedures are outlined here, we want to emphasize that it is the *spirit* of the endeavour that counts, not the letter of the law. What we are pursuing here is a health promotion approach that is empowering, under community control, and which enhances the health, well-being, quality of life and spiritual strength of people in a positive and culturally appropriate way. How it is done is a matter of taste, personality, local situation and cultural setting. So, please, as you read the following, keep the broad picture in mind, even though at times we might seem to get into quite exact details. The reason for being detailed from time to time is simply to show that it *can* be done—that these "noble" principles can actually be translated into real living situations, and be of benefit in those situations.

9

APPLYING PCHP PRINCIPLES
General Considerations and Introduction to the People System

To do what we want to do here, it would be preferable to be interacting with you, the reader, in a workshop kind of format. The ideal would be for you to bring along the issues, ideas, problems or situations you are most interested in, and then we could discuss how you could apply the principles we have been talking about. What we *have* done is to use drafts of this book in situations with students and practitioners over several years, and have tried to adapt what we have written here to what arose in those situations. So we hope what you find here can be related to what interests you.

The initial step when faced with a new situation, or trying to plan a piece of research or an intervention, is always to go back to first principles. So what are the first principles when actually beginning to start on, or think about, a new project?

Principle Number One is to attempt to *see the issue from the perspective of the people concerned*. For example, maybe you have been asked to do something about a problem of glue-sniffing at the local high school. No doubt everyone has a theory as to why this is a problem, and there may be truth in many of those theories. The teachers probably have a pretty good idea of what is going on, and can probably give quite a good social analysis of the situation. For example, it is likely that the kids concerned are underachievers, come from backgrounds of educational or material lack, have low self-esteem, may be being abused at home, etc. etc. They may be of certain ethnic, cultural or other identifiable subgroups. All these things are relevant, but they are not an explanation. The only way one can really get to the heart of the matter is to find out how the kids themselves see themselves and the world they live in. Whether one can get these students to talk at all is an issue—but with the right people to do the talking with them, that will probably only be a temporary problem. Most kids talk readily when they trust and respect someone. So, how *do* they see the world? Are they the dumb, no-hopers that some might portray them as? One thing that most of us find when we *do* talk to the people that the official services often label as "hopeless" or "stupid" is that they are neither of those things. As we start to understand them in a "compassionate" way (get our own egos, opinions and prejudices out of the way), we can start to get a feel of what is going on, and what worthwhile human beings we are dealing with, even if on the surface they might look otherwise. We assert that it is only by this "radical subjectivity", by allowing the people concerned to voice their deepest perceptions, world views, and feelings about themselves and their situation, that the "truth" will emerge. And it is this "truth" on which action should be based— not on one's ego-based judgements, or some other "outsider's" view. And, here, even the parents of the children in our example are likely to be outsiders. For example, in one PCHP project, the organizers were struck by the disparity between survey results coming from parents of teenagers about what they thought their teenagers needed in the way of community facilities and activities, and what those same teenagers said themselves. It was as though two entirely separate universes had been sampled. So even those who are theoretically knowledgeable about a particular social group cannot necessarily speak for those people—only the people themselves can. So Principle Number One involves allowing the people of concern to speak for themselves, and attempting to understand them in those terms, without one's own emotions, thoughts and opinions clouding the picture. We would bet that just doing this would start to make the appropriate action emerge out of the "fog" of possibilities. And, of course, the people concerned can be asked what they think is the best action to take about a situation, and their ideas on what to do are likely to be as good as anyone else's, and probably better.

Principle Number Two is to *remind ourselves about the philosophy*. Above all, the key concept here is *empowerment*. Let us suppose that we have been invited into a town where there is high unemployment and much health and mental health related distress associated with this situation. Let us also suppose that we think we could get a research grant to study the situation, and maybe undertake a "demonstration project" to show what could be done. Perhaps we have some pretty good ideas about the directions this could take. How then would one proceed in an empowering way? What would be a disempowering way to go? Without reading further, why not think about or discuss these questions for a moment or two. Okay, what did you come up with?

A disempowering way to proceed would, for example, be to go away and write a research proposal without consulting the community, and apply for funds. Maybe one might talk to one's colleagues, and one or two people in the community. But no wide-scale consultation.

A slightly more empowering approach would be to talk with a number of key people in the community, and then write the proposal.

Even more empowering would be to have widespread discussions with many people in the community and, in particular, with those most affected by the unemployment. You would enter into a relationship of "radical subjectivity" with them, getting their views, sounding them out about possibilities, seeing whether they are interested in "doing something", and so on. At this stage, this is not "systematic research", nor should it be. (This is prior to actually undertaking a project, remember.) But it is getting a feel for the community, and where people are at. This process would also help to identify potential resource people in the community, who could later undertake organizational roles.

Even more empowering still would be to do everything that is contained in the previous paragraph, but be committed as well to the concept of community control. That is, if the project is to proceed at all, while it may need your expertise as a researcher to help to get it up and running, the control of the project has to be in the hands of the community. This immediately brings up the question of organizational mechanisms for enabling such community control to happen. As will be seen, our view is that it is usually best to start with an organization that addresses itself specifically to the matters in hand, rather than trying to graft the project on to an existing body or interest group. Too often, existing bodies have their own agendas, already-committed resources, and general "baggage". A new organization permits one to build in PCHP principles, which are not the typical principles by which most organizations run, community or otherwise. In our experience, the model of the "incorporated society" is a good one—that is, a grouping that has a legal existence, and which has a constitution and set of objectives specifically designed to uphold the principles of empowerment and PCHP philosophy within that organization. To summarize the point we are making: the principle of empowerment in a community project means ultimately to have the control of that project unambiguously in the hands of the people of concern. This is, of course, only one (although very important) manifestation of the empowerment principle in a project—others we will cover later.

Other PCHP philosophical principles need to be remembered at this early stage too—the need for good organization, the commitment to needs assessment as we define it here (systematically or representatively finding out what people want for themselves), a facilitating way of working (with regard both to experts who work with the community, and to the way community people work with themselves), a positive approach to problem-solving (we say more about this in a moment), and an ecological or global approach (which we also look at in a moment). We also believe that there should be an early commitment to evaluation and clear goals. All these matters need to be in one's head as one proceeds, even at this very early stage.

Another important "philosophical principle" is to ensure that, if you have come into a situation to tackle a "problem" such as suicide, smoking, drugs, sexual abuse, deaths from heart disease, the stresses of having a sick child, unemployment, depression, racial oppression, bad housing, etc., all of which are framed negatively, you then attempt to see if it can be *reframed positively*. Certainly, there is a need to know realistically what the problems are, and one would want to monitor the impact of any project on them. But having got that clear, the art then becomes one of "lifting the tone" by seeing if the problems can be addressed positively. That is, can one work on the problems in a *strength-building* way, not a "problem-fixing" way? This is, of course, just a variation on the theme of empowerment. We see, in PCHP, that the key to the solution of human problems is to reframe things so that these problems are dealt with as part of an enterprise that is positive, strength-building and supportive. This approach is one that seeks to identify existing assets, then builds on those, on the terms of the people involved. Here, we accept the view that virtually all people, no matter how violent, stressed, ill or dispossessed, have the wish and capacity for wellness, health, sanity and balance. All we need to do as professionals or facilitators is to set up the conditions for those things to emerge naturally, and they will. So the strengths that are being "built" are the strengths that were there all the time—they were just being masked by circumstances, stresses, lack of opportunity, resentments, oppression, etc. Given the right environment, they will come to the fore, and the "health" that emerges is simply an expression of what was already there in nascent form.

This then brings us to Principle Number Three—that of taking a *generic, holistic or ecological approach*. In some respects, this is the hardest of all for people in the helping services to grasp, partly since most funding or employing agencies do not think this way. Not only are most of the "problems" that trigger health promotion or community action typically framed negatively, but they are also typically very focused. For example, only a few days ago, someone called one of us to ask if we could be involved in a project to reduce smoking in a certain ethnic group. Our immediate response was, "How can we reframe that issue so that (a) it is a positive strength-building project, and (b) it can be viewed in its wider context?"

So what exactly do we mean here? Typically, as we say, health promoters are asked to address a specific, negative issue—smoking, sexual abuse, AIDS, teenage suicide, etc. Certainly, one can get some mileage out of a frontal attack on the "problem". However, what we favour is a more generic, positive, developmental approach. We need to see the "problem" in its wider context. That is, if smoking is a problem in a certain age group of a certain ethnic group, what is going on there? If sexual abuse is occurring in certain identifiable groups in certain geographical areas, what is going on there?

Connected to this is also the propensity to divide the world into "target groups". We have already had something to say about this, but we will say it again here. Too often, we see "community" being divided into "women", "men", "teenagers", "the unemployed", "the poor", "the disabled", "the elderly", etc. etc. We do not deny that each of these groupings has its own characteristics, needs and issues. However, to abstract them from the wider community context is, in our view, not the way to proceed. This is one reason why we prefer a locality-based community approach. The usual way of cutting a population down to a manageable size for an intervention is to define it in terms of a "problem". However, this raises all the issues we have just alluded to—of negativity, of isolation from wider community process, and so on. The *other* way to reduce the size of a population is to limit its geographical size, but then to include everyone who is in that geographical area.

We are aware of many of the conventional objections to this. Some say we cannot easily define a community by its boundaries. Others assert that we should not include everyone in a community, because this will deflect attention from the "most needy". That is, if we include everyone in a mixed community, the "privileged" or "middle class" will grab all the resources, and the "underprivileged" will get forgotten again. In our view, the opposite is what can be true. Most communities can define their own actual or potential boundaries. And provided the situation is handled properly, and one is constantly aware of the dangers of a "middle class takeover" (or some equivalent), then the considerable strengths and resources that the "middle class" or privileged group can bring to a community endeavour can often be harnessed to the benefit of all. This embodies an important philosophical principle. Our view of community is one that is whole, organic and "natural". To divide it up along "problem" or "target group" lines is simply to perpetuate the fragmentation and divisiveness that already characterize and damage much of our world. Instead, if we can seek constructive ways to operate together in harmony, so that the strengths of everyone are used to the benefit of all, we believe this is a superior mode. It is the one we pursue here, while being aware of its intrinsic difficulties.

Principle Number Four, and the final one here, is that of *evaluation*. This in turn is strongly linked to the principle of *needs assessment*, which we mentioned earlier as vital to a PCHP approach. Evaluation is often thought about at the end of a project rather than in its early stages. Yet, if evaluation is built in at the outset, the whole enterprise can be shaped in evaluative terms. Not only does this assist later evaluation, but more importantly it is an optimal way to plan the whole mode of operating. To begin with, the kind of evaluation we favour is oriented around goals. Goals are a formulation of the *positive* tasks one wants to undertake to make the project proceed optimally. In short, goals are positivity operationalized. Goals, in turn, make it imperative that one is very clear about *needs*. Now, "needs" is a tricky term, and we talk more about it later. However, as mentioned above, what *we* mean by "needs" is the articulation by the people of concern about what they want for themselves. It is the expression of their "deep subjectivity", in terms of (once it is clear what a project is generally about, and people have bought into the concept) what it is that the project can do for them, and for their community. The goals are the translation into action of deeply felt wishes, that come from the hearts and vision of the people themselves. Of course, it is not a straightforward process to get a representative picture of needs, and it is an art to sort these into positive action in an orderly way that still appeals to the community. But it certainly can be done, and the best approach is a participatory one. (We will spend quite a lot of time on this later.) The whole basis of PCHP in practice involves the ascertaining of genuine, self-expressed needs, the translation of these into practical, clear, positive goals, the basing of action on these goals, and the evaluation of whether the goals have been accomplished and needs have successfully been met. This in turn requires a continuous process of review and critical appraisal, relating both to whether things are on track, and to whether things seem to be working. This is at the heart of the evaluation enterprise. Evaluation serves both to assess outcomes, and to keep the whole show on the road. Above all, what is desirable in any project is the development of a climate of positive self-criticism, of wanting to know why things are not going better, and why we went wrong, so that we can do it better next time.

THE PEOPLE SYSTEM

The People System is "PCHP in action". It is a procedural model that takes PCHP principles, and turns them into a step-by-step way of going about things that ensures those principles are fully realized—or at least to the extent that a given situation allows. The rest of this book is largely about how to apply PCHP principles using the People System.

The model is one that has been developed by John Raeburn over a 20-year period in New Zealand, and also in Canada under the name "People Projects" (Raeburn, 1987). It is close to what in Canada is called the "planning model". But its special feature is the attempt to incorporate everything we have been talking about so far into a single operational system.

In this context, the term "People" still continues to mean what was covered in Chapter 2 as the mnemonic for People System principles. But, in addition, it is also an acronym for "*P*lanning and *E*valuation *O*f *P*eople-*L*ed *E*ndeavours". At the heart of People System projects is *community control*, which is, as we have said, the pivotal concept for empowering approaches to health promotion. Hence the phrase "People-Led Endeavours". The

"Planning and Evaluation" part of the acronym signifies the other important emphasis, which is a systematic and planned approach, centred around the concept of evaluation. *Goals* and *needs/wishes assessments* are a crucial part of the evaluation approach used here. As for the term "System", what we have adopted here is a "systems" approach in at least three senses of that term.

First, an overall inspiration for this sort of approach is General System Theory, originated by Ludwig von Bertalanffy (von Bertalanffy, 1968). This is not the time to go into von Bertalanffy's work in detail. In brief, what he says is that the whole of nature (he was a biologist) and the universe consists of systems, which are defined as "sets of elements standing in interrelation". "General system theory . . . is a general science of wholeness." Whereas in the past, science has tended to analyse things in a vacuum, finding it easier to reduce complex wholes to their simpler components, reality is actually structured in terms of wholes, and these wholes are more than their individual component parts. Such considerations become especially relevant when we come to complex biological systems like people, and complex social systems like communities and nations. For example, it is customary in most medical thinking to reduce people to their constituent organ systems, bones, limbs or other parts. However, these "component parts" only exist realistically as a part of a greater context or "truth", and it is often silly to abstract them from these interconnections. We could pursue these matters for the rest of this book, but perhaps even these brief comments show why, in considering topics like health, people, culture and community, a "systems" view is applicable.

Von Bertalanffy had many interesting things to say about systems. One is that they obey laws like anything else in nature. What is true for one system is usually true for another of similar type. For example, most systems have a "stasis", a dynamic equilibrium that holds the system in its present form. Inputs to the system threaten its stasis, and put it into disequilibrium or "stress". The system then usually acts to bring things back to where they were (as in "homeostasis"). As a result, most systems are seen as being resistant to change, something we, as those who work with people, are usually only too aware of, regardless of whether the systems are individuals, institutions or whole communities. However, systems do change gradually in response to constant inputs (as an ecosystem like a lake can change through, say, silting up), and most systems do have a "threshold" where, in response to inputs of sufficient strength, they will go into disequilibrium, until they re-form around a new stasis, which takes the new "reality" into account. We trust it can be seen that this way of looking at things can be useful for the community development and health promotion worker.

A second way the People System uses the concept of "system" is as a procedural approach, as represented by writers such as Churchman (1968). That is, there is a set of operations associated with "systems analysis" and system change which follow steps such as needs assessment, goal-setting, review of processes, and so on. This kind of approach is indeed widely used in business and institutions, and is the basis of organizational development. "Community organization" on the American model falls into this category. The People System also follows this sort of procedural model. Here, the procedures are laid down in a relatively predictable, chronological or logical sequence, and are followed through in a systematic way. At the heart of this process are goals, which are the organizational units around which the procedures are built.

The third use of the term "system" relates to what are sometimes called "cybernetics" or "control" systems. This is where a system is deliberately set up to meet certain goals. A cybernetics system is one that not only has goals aimed at taking it in a certain direction, but which also has built in "review" and "feedback" processes, so that there is constant monitoring of whether the system is "on track" for meeting its goals. An illustration that is often used, though not an especially palatable one, is of a missile launched with a target set into its internal computer. Because of wind and other factors, a missile may deviate periodically from its flight path. The internal "review" systems detect this deviation, and instantly correct the flight path back on target. If the missile is on target when the check is made, its current direction is confirmed. The first review procedure, where a deviation is detected and corrected, involves what is called "negative feedback"—that is, a negativity is detected and "information" is transmitted to the control mechanisms to correct it. The second, where the existing direction is confirmed, is called "positive feedback". These terms have come into the common language, but this particular usage in a cybernetics framework is useful to remember. As will be seen in our subsequent discussions of the procedures involved in applying the People System, ongoing review processes are an intrinsic part of those procedures and central to them. "Errors" (that is, goals that are not being attained, or other things not happening as they might) are detected as they happen, and immediate action is taken to correct them, in a supportive rather than punitive atmosphere. *Any* system has its deviations from the "flight path". People working in the system can see such deviations or "errors" as an opportunity for problem-solving on a group basis, then taking corrective action and learning from this. When review procedures show that things are on track, this is an opportunity for "positive feedback" (such as the explicit acknowledgement of someone's good work). It is good for the morale of the whole organization to know when things are going well, which is usually most of the time. What we have, then, is a "system" (a project or other undertaking) that is self-optimizing and capable of producing and maintaining high morale. This, we believe, is a very good way for any system to go.

This discussion of systems is, admittedly, very short, and we hope you will feel interested enough to find out more. However, we trust it is enough to show why we think this is a good approach.

To summarize, then, the People System is an approach to planning, running and evaluating health promotion projects that incorporate the values and principles of PCHP. It is a systematic procedural approach, and puts considerable emphasis on empowerment and community control. It is probably most suitable for larger scale community projects. However, as will be seen from the examples, it can actually be used with projects ranging from individual client programmes, through small group activities, to community projects involving whole communities or regions. In Chapter 10, we will look at the general steps involved in using the People System.

10

THE PEOPLE SYSTEM
A General Guide

In this chapter, we look at the steps involved in setting up a project on the People System model. It will be noted that we are using the term "project", which *The Concise Oxford Dictionary* (1984) defines as "scheme, planned undertaking"—that is, a planned enterprise of some substance. Here, the aim is to show, based on actual experience, how this kind of approach is taken in practice. The "project" we have chosen is of a generic, locality-based, community-development type, but we hope that this example will serve to show how to proceed not only with a project like this, but with other types as well. (Descriptions of a variety of actual applications are provided in Chapters 12–14.)

We cover the procedures by listing 13 steps to follow in establishing and running a project. The style used is a set of recommendations to you, the reader, on the assumption you are a community worker who is involved in setting up and facilitating a project. We hope these steps are equally usable by professionals and non-professionals, although most readers are likely to be the former, and we assume that perspective.

Step 1: Begin an Initial Consultation about the Concept of the Project

The first thing that usually needs to happen with any project is a get-together of the interested parties to map out what is wanted, and to agree on the overall philosophy. This latter step is not usually a part of many community activities, but is crucial here. As can already be seen, PCHP is heavy on philosophy, by which we mean values, overall vision and an agreed-on way of working.

Who, then, are the "interested parties" that might get together to discuss a project in the initial phases? This question is absolutely vital, and has to do with who initiates an idea, and how the initiators are going to relate to the "community of interest".

At this stage, we need to get at least one term clear—that is, "community of interest" (COI). Here, we use this term to refer specifically to those people, at the community level, who are most affected by, and interested in, the project. Presumably all health promotion projects have intended beneficiaries. The aim is the improvement of health, well-being, quality of life, or some other such thing of a group of people. That is the COI, as we define it here. But what is crucial, following a PCHP approach, is that the COI are also the *planners, controllers and principal actors in the project*. For this discussion, most of the time we assume that the COI is a locality-based community. That is, it is identified with a specific location. Our view is that the ideal size of a "community" for working in this way is between 5000 and 10 000 people. However, a COI could range anywhere from being a small group up to being, say, 300 000 people.

Now, to return to a vital question—who is initiating this project? In particular, has the initiative come from the COI, or from some outside person or agency?

Ideally, the impulse for a project should come from within the community itself, and there is no doubt that, when this happens, it is more likely to be successful. To be realistic, however, many if not most health promotion projects will have their seeds in some idea, policy, plan or suggestion that comes from outside the COI. For example, there are many health or other agencies around with an overview of the situation in various communities, and they will perceive a problem or supposed need. Or, alternatively, a student may want to do a research project, sees a likely community in which to undertake that project, and then will want to get started.

Let us, then, take this less than optimal situation where some outside agency or person wants to undertake something in a community with a perceived need, but where there has been no particular expression of interest from that community about having such a project.

First of all, the way to proceed here is, we believe, with great sensitivity. We need to be aware of all the potential pitfalls of coming into a community with a preconceived idea. Second, if we do think we have something to offer that is important and beneficial for that community, then we had better start checking that out with the community right away. That is, we need to talk with people in the community to see if there is a general feeling of support for what is proposed. Again, this is following the principle of being guided by people's subjectivity. It is *their* view of the matter in hand, and *their* emotional reaction to it, that counts. Either it grabs their hearts and minds, or it doesn't. The wise worker has to sift through the different reactions, and come to a conclusion about whether to proceed with the original idea, modify it, or scrap it.

At this early stage, it may be appropriate not only to talk to key members of the COI as individuals, but also to hold meetings of interested groups. Often, at such meetings, one can start to get more of a collective feel of where the community is at. Also, people often feel able to voice stronger objections in a meeting, than if you see them face to face. Again, such meetings are not necessarily representative of everyone's view, but they will give a good overall flavour of what the community is about, and how they are likely to take to what is being proposed.

With this initial consultation phase behind you, and confident that the community is keen about what is being proposed, you are ready to move on to the next step, or the next two steps—starting to set up a community grouping of people to administer and run the project, and doing a more formal survey of wishes and needs.

Step 2: Set up the Initial Organization

If the community has initiated the action, then we already have a group to relate to. But if it is us who are getting things going, then the next step is to organize a small or not so small group of community people with whom to have continuing discussions, and who will evolve into an enduring group to carry the future organizational responsibility.

Hopefully, the initial consultation will have thrown up one or two or more people who are especially interested in what is going on. Ideally, these people will include someone who has organizational skills, and someone with "people skills".

This core group serves a number of purposes. First, they provide a forum for an exchange of ideas about philosophy, objectives and general strategy. Second, they provide local community continuity for the project. However, if there is currently no one from the community who can take on a leadership role, but you are able to, you may find for a while that this is necessary. However, your agenda is always to find someone who can take over from you, and for whom you may be a guide or "model" until they have learned the skills to do what you can do. This embodies a vital principle for leadership roles in a community project—that of facilitation, sharing skills, fading and back-up. That is, if someone (which may be you) has skills that others do not have, then the aim is to share those skills around as much as possible. To begin with (if it is you), you may do the job (e.g. coordinating some activity). Then you look for someone who could potentially learn those same skills, and be good in the job. You then transmit those skills, mainly through modelling plus instruction. (A written manual for complex tasks is also sometimes useful.) Once you are confident the person has the requisite skills, you let them do the job, and once they can operate independently, "fade" yourself until you are no longer around. However, you tell the person you are available for support, if need be, on the end of a phone or by some other means. Finally, of course, they will not even need this prop in most cases. This is a model we have used for many years in various community projects, and it seems to contain many of the essential elements of empowerment, in that it leads to the development of important skills by many people; the inference is that most people can learn to be a leader. (However, not everyone can be all types of leader—some are better with people, others with "business"-type activities, and so on. So the fitting of people to appropriate leadership roles is important here too.)

This "steering group" may function for quite a long period of time. Eventually, of course, it will be time to set up the more long-term organizational structure, and we deal with this in Step 5. All the time, however, the vision of being open to community input, continuous consultation, and so on, is important, so that this group does not become a "clique" from which others feel excluded. It will be important to keep the community, and interested parties in the community, informed of what is going on, and to be aware of the public relations side of what is happening generally.

This raises the question of the media and publicity for what is going on. Often, if something exciting is happening, the media may hear of it and want to write a story on it. Here, you will have to use your judgement. In general, the secret is to use the media to your advantage, rather than just have them do a story for its own sake. For example, if you are about to do a survey, then it may be advantageous to have the community know about what is coming, and a media story could accomplish this. On the other hand, one does not necessarily want community expectations raised unduly by a premature release of plans, or for the community to find out vital information from the media, when they should have found out directly through other means.

Also relevant here is the question of other bodies in the community with a stake in what is being planned. It is very easy, with the arrival of a new project, especially if it is of relatively major proportions, for other bodies to feel threatened. Strenuous efforts will need to be made to see that this does not occur, which may mean quite a lot of time spent talking to people in those bodies, going to meetings, etc. In general, on the basis of the "cohesion-building" model of community we espouse, the aim is the co-operative working together of all bodies in a community. If the proposed project is likely to relate to, or cover the same ground as, another activity or organization in the community, then great tact is required, and you will need to give credible assurances to those people that your plans are to facilitate their work, not cut across it.

It is probably clear now why this initial phase of planning and development of the organization takes time. Not only do the ideas need to be sorted out, discussed and solidified, but many people have to be consulted, appeased, informed, and so on. Ideas and input need to be sought all the time, so that there emerges a feeling of ownership of, and goodwill towards, what is being proposed on the part of the wider community.

Step 3: Organize a Needs Assessment

Needs assessment, as defined in a People System context, means ascertaining what people want for themselves. This stands in contrast to the prevailing health system philosophy of professionals deciding what is good for people. In the People System approach, the philosophy is one of people making their own decisions about what is good for them, and then having all action flow from that.

We feel that the premium instrument for needs assessment is the well-executed random survey, although other methods are important too. The major advantage of the survey is that it is *representative*. What the random sample survey does is ensure a voice for everyone in the COI and, provided the sampling is done well, one should get a real "cross-section". In particular, this ensures that those who do not normally speak up at meetings, or would not necessarily get the opportunity to say anything, are heard. It also means that the multiple voices in a community are heard in proportion to their presence in that whole community, rather than just the voices of those who are well organized, articulate, or who otherwise might get the ear of the planners.

Now, it is agreed that surveys may not provide much depth of information. Also, they may not always be culturally appropriate. Certainly, one may have to adapt surveys to the cultural context in which they are done, and have them executed by peers in that culture. What is important is that the general principles being enunciated here are observed. That is, the information-gathering needs to be democratic and empowering, which means that everyone in the community has an equal say, and every effort is made to get input from those who may not normally be heard.

There are many variations on survey methodology and content. We do not wish to go into these here. However, it is worth saying just one or two things about these aspects.

First, whenever possible, it is important to construct any survey in ongoing consultation with the COI.

Second, needs-assessment surveys do not have to be too long, time-consuming or expensive. That is, it is not usually necessary to have samples of the same size as in other types of surveys, such as political opinion surveys. We are basically after an impressionistic (though accurate) picture of the needs, wishes and suggestions of the community, in some sort of prioritized form, which will aid the process of planning and goal-setting.

Third, it is very important to be clear about the objectives of the survey, and to design each question to fit those objectives. The main aim of a survey in a People System context is to find out what people want in relation to a domain of interest, so that specific goals can then be set in the project to meet these wishes.

Fourth, although the survey is structured or semi-structured, there needs to be ample opportunity for including and recording ancillary qualitative information.

What we are aiming for, then, is both science and art. Ultimately, the needs-assessment process, as we have characterized it here, is to provide the information needed to plan and implement action. We also want to capture the spirit of what people want in a community, so that it will draw them into participation in a "magnetic" way. Certainly, we believe at a very profound level, that *needs assessment of this type is the key, the secret, to successful community development action*, simply because it grasps what people really want for themselves, so that it is their deeply felt wishes that are driving the project.

Step 4: Prioritize Needs and Set Goals

Once the survey has been analysed, there will be raw data showing, say, percentages of support and ideas for different needs, wishes and strategies for action. The task now is to order this list in terms of priorities. This requires combining the actual frequencies from the survey data with more qualitative information, and with general knowledge about the community and the resources that are available. The best way to proceed here is, as far as possible, to prioritize needs and set goals in a collaborative, consultative way, involving as many people from the COI as is practicable.

Our own preference, in a project of any size that is likely to go on for some years, has been to have goal-setting based on 12-month periods. That is, the main operational goals are "annual goals". Annual goals occupy a position intermediate between long-term goals, for example five-year goals, and short-term goals—what needs to be done on a week-to-week or month-to-month basis to meet the annual goals. (These short-term goals we call "working goals".)

The setting of clearly stated, time-limited goals has, we believe, great value. They focus people's minds on exactly what it is the project is about, and how the philosophy and needs are going to be translated into actual action. The goals give direction, in that they specify, when well written, a concrete target or desirable outcome to have been reached by a set date. The *writing down* of goals is very important. This constitutes a formal acceptance of the goals, stated in clear language, and means they can be communicated readily to anyone and everyone. All action flows from these goals, and they should be kept visible and prominent at all times.

Goals mean that things keep on track, and are not subverted by "good ideas" that come along, say, in the middle of the goal year. Inevitably, community projects are tempted to go off track to accommodate some new circumstance or supposed priority that may come up during the year. (Such new priorities, if they are important, can be incorporated into the *next* annual goal exercise.)

Goals provide a basic organizational unit, in the sense that the activities or subprojects that constitute the main operations of the project can each take an annual goal as its driving force. Or to put it around the other way, an annual goal would lead to the setting up of a subproject or organized activity aimed at meeting that goal. This also gives an idea as to the "size" of an annual goal. In some community projects, for example, we have had a broad rule of thumb that about a dozen annual goals is the right number. This means there would be 12 or so different projects or activity areas under the umbrella of an overall community development project. Each of those projects would then have a "convener" associated with it, and this person would then organize others to help. In short, then, the overall organization is really a set of subprojects, each with its own annual goal driving it, and each with its own convener responsible for seeing that a particular goal is attained.

Goals also play a central role in evaluation. They can be used as the basis for the ongoing internal review processes (see Step 11). And if they are written properly, they can be used for "outcome evaluation" at the end of the year by determining whether or not they have been attained (see Chapter 11).

Finally, the advantage of goals is that they represent a *positive* expression of *practical action* that can be taken to meet needs. They cast the whole undertaking into positive, do-able chunks, and this in turn creates its own positive energy.

Thus *the use of goals as a basic organizational tool in this kind of health promotion is highly recommended.*

Our experience is that it takes time to set up a goal system in a community-based project. However, once a "goal culture" is established, everyone seems to like the use of goals, even though they may have initially resisted their use.

Step 5: Start Thinking about Changing from a Steering Group to a More Permanent Organizational Structure

Although for ease of presentation we have put this step after the goal-setting process, what we are talking about here could happen at almost any time. Certainly, at some stage, the steering committee will have to examine the whole organizational issue, and there will come a time when it is appropriate to act.

As mentioned previously, one structure for setting up a community project of any scale is the incorporated society. This provides a vehicle by which an organization can be given legal standing in the community, and which makes it "respectable" and "real". Its advantages for our purposes are that (a) it requires the group to state its objectives clearly (the objectives have to be put into the constitution), (b) it requires the setting up of an elected committee to run things, and (c) it means that the money and resource management are audited and generally put into an accountable framework. Above all, however, the merit of the incorporated society framework is that it establishes a *new* body, which is autonomous and totally committed to the project in hand, rather than being grafted on to another body, or being part of a bureaucracy. *It means that the community, via its elected committee, is in control, not some other body or organization.*

Step 6: Re-examine the Philosophy and Objectives

By the time the steering group has got round to changing to a more permanent organizational structure, they will have "lived with" the philosophy and principles with which they started, and will have a better feel for these. The writing of constitutional objectives is a good moment to re-examine the original statements, and to revisit what the philosophy is, and what the organization is trying to achieve. What one requires, at this stage, is an essential consensus about how to do things. One reason this is necessary is that keeping things goal-oriented and empowering is often contrary to the inclinations of some participants. Therefore it is important further down the track, when these principles may be under strain, to know that the philosophy was arrived at through a consensual process involving all major players and the community.

This philosophy, couched in terms of objectives, could cover such matters as:

- to be concerned with, and attempt to enhance, the health, well-being and quality of life of the community of interest
- to emphasize community-building and a sense of community
- to do this in a way that is empowering, positive and strength-building
- to base all action on representatively ascertained needs and wishes
- to be involved with all sectors of the community, young and old, rich and poor, male and female, all ethnic and cultural groups, etc.
- to be committed to principles of cultural awareness, cultural safety, and the valuing of cultural diversity, and to upholding whatever treaty or culturally relevant legal obligations there might be in that setting
- to give special emphasis to the needs of those who might otherwise miss out
- to be committed to the evaluation of all processes and outcomes

Obviously, this is only a very general statement of objectives, and each individual case would have its own variations and additions. But it gives a flavour of the kind of thing that can be said.

Step 7: Work out the Relationship between the Committee/Board and the Staff

Most projects will have a committee or board to oversee them, and may have paid or unpaid staff. The relationship between these two components of the organization requires some thinking about. If the staff are paid, the committee would be the employer, and would have to meet the requirements of being a "good" employer, which may include such things as contracts, accident insurance, conflict resolution, and so on. This may sound a bit complicated, but at least it makes the formal relationship between the committee and the staff clear, and the staff are indisputably answerable to the committee for what they do. The situation is not so clear, however, when the staff are largely or wholly voluntary. Here, it is more difficult to work out how the two sides relate to each other, especially since it is likely that committee members will also be doing voluntary activities within the broader organization. In a voluntary situation, it may also be more difficult for philosophies to be policed in any effective way, since so much is dependent on the goodwill of people, and the retention of informal community relationships.

Various arrangements are possible, and none seems perfect. Our suggestion is that the following is a generally appropriate breakdown of powers:

Committee
- keep an overview of the whole operation and are guardians of the overall philosophy
- are watchdogs on behalf of the community-at-large
- provide continuity over time, when workers might come and go
- are responsible for broad policy decisions (as resolutions), but take these decisions on the advice of the workers, and generally attempt to work in harmony with workers, to facilitate their action
- are responsible for obtaining and managing the money, facilities and other material resources required to run the operation
- through the Chair, are responsible for resolving conflicts and other worker issues that threaten the well-being of the whole organization
- are the employer when workers are paid

Staff
- are responsible for organizing and executing needs assessment and evaluation processes

- are responsible for finding, training and supporting leaders of activities, and for generally dealing with the people resources required to run the operation
- are responsible for coordinating activities and programmes on a day-to-day basis
- are responsible for organizing education activities within the project, and for liaison and public relations with other bodies and organizations, both inside and outside the community

Step 8: Do a Resource-planning Exercise

The term "resources" in this context primarily means money for a variety of purposes. However, many projects will also need facilities such as a centre, and equipment of various kinds. Expertise may also be another requirement, and this might have to be bought or otherwise obtained on a consultancy basis, or through educational materials. Support and goodwill from other agencies in the community and other bodies outside the community may also be required or desirable. However, the most important resource is people—community people who are prepared to participate, and take on a range of roles.

Of all these resource areas, money is probably the most difficult to get. This is not the place to go into detail about all the options that a community project might explore to seek funding, but these might include grants, local fund-raising, commercial operations associated with the project, adult education teacher-funding to pay trainers, local government support, health authority support or salaries, business sponsorship, door-to-door collections, local economic development, and so on. Usually, most projects will have to rely on multiple funding sources, rather than a single one.

Of all the resource decisions that need to be made, perhaps the most important has to do with whether or not workers will be paid. It is difficult to generalize across projects, but our view is that, on the whole, a project is more likely to succeed if key people can be paid. This is because it allows one to get and retain the best people for leadership roles in the project. That is, the most talented people in a community are always in demand and, if one is to secure and hold them, money is a help! (As a rule of thumb, we have found that the amount of voluntary time one can expect most people to offer is about three to four hours a week.) Almost all voluntary activity has some costs associated with it for the individual. These costs could be financial, such as running a car. Or they could be social, such as time away from one's family. In either case, some financial acknowledgement is helpful. In the family example, sometimes a spouse might resent the time the other person is putting into a voluntary endeavour, and some form of payment shows the value to the household of this work.

Step 9: Work out Worker Requirements and Guidelines

In a large community project, it may be helpful to have two rather than just one "coordinator". One reason for this is that it avoids having the whole responsibility and focus invested on one person—two part-time people are generally better here than one full-time person. Also, a wide range of skills is required to be a successful coordinator of a complex community project, and it may be unrealistic to think one person would have them all. One arrangement that has worked well is to have one coordinator responsible for the "people" side (finding people to fill roles and seeing that these people have the skills and support to do what needs to be done), and to have a second coordinator responsible for the planning and evaluation systems (she or he is a "systems manager" rather than a direct "people person"). Because the needs assessment, goal-setting, review, evaluation, guideline-writing and other such processes are so vital, but also take a lot of time, especially initially, the project needs to show its commitment to these things by making a senior person responsible for them.

It is usually helpful to have all procedures written down, and all major roles summarized in a set of guidelines. Not only does this translate "lessons" learned by individuals into a form from which others can benefit, but even more importantly, it makes the job roles transcend the particular individuals who occupy them. The reality is that there is always turnover of people, and the less dependent a position is on one person who has all the knowledge in his or her head, the better.

Step 10: Plan and Set up Subprojects to Meet Annual Goals

Now we come to the heartland of "taking action" within the project. Suppose that the needs-assessment process has led to the setting of 10 annual goals, prioritized in rank order from 1 to 10, and all with the same deadline 12 months hence. These might read something like:

By 1 December (next year):

1. To have found a centre from which to organize this project, and which can serve as a meeting place for people in the community.
2. To have set up a childcare facility so that parents can be free of their children for a few hours during the day, to take part in community activities.

continues

— continued —

3. To have available a range of at least five different job-skills acquisition workshops, with a special focus on those who are unemployed.
4. To have started at least two lifestyle health programmes in accordance with the priorities shown in the survey, in particular for weight control and healthy eating, and possibly exercise.

. . . and so on.

Each of these is quite a major undertaking, and what is envisaged here is that each annual goal would have a convener who is in charge of seeing that it is accomplished. This goal-oriented action component is what we are calling a subproject.

Step 11: Establish Goal-setting and Review Meetings

This step is of fundamental importance to the successful operation of a project of this nature, with so many people working on so many different tasks. It is at the heart of the project as a "cybernetics system"—that is, a system where progress towards attaining goals is constantly monitored, with positive or negative feedback occurring as a consequence.

The term "goal-setting and review meeting" (GSR meeting) indicates that such meetings combine these two functions. These meetings involve the conveners of all subprojects and should probably take place once a week, or certainly once every two weeks. At meetings, annual goals are considered one by one in terms of "working goals" set at each such meeting. These working goals break the annual goals down into successive and concrete tasks, which are realistically able to be done in a week, or whatever the review period is. For example, a working goal for the childcare facility annual goal listed above could be: "By the next GSR meeting, to have investigated possible locations for setting up a facility". Such goals would be set at each GSR meeting.

The other component of the GSR meeting—review—is simply for the relevant convener to report on whether or not the working goal or goals have been achieved.

All this has to be done in a systematic way, and the role of a facilitator or Chair for these meetings is vital. This needs to be a person who can confidently keep everyone to the rules of the meeting. In particular, she or he needs to be able to stop irrelevant discussion in a way that is positive and friendly! The system collapses as soon as it is felt that these GSR meetings are out of control, too long, or too boring. It is suggested that, once a good GSR meeting facilitator is found, that person should keep the job, since it is a skill that not everyone has!

One other crucial point needs to be made here. The GSR meeting has an important part to play for the whole morale and ethos of a project. It is probably the most regular occasion on which all the key players in a project will get together. Also, the response of the meeting to "successes" and "failures" when working-goal progress is being reported on is a powerful force in a project. Generally, such a meeting will respond with spontaneous positivity to goals achieved, which is very "reinforcing" for those who have worked hard on those goals. On the other hand, if difficulties have been encountered, and a goal has not been achieved, the ethos to be aimed at is one of friendly and supportive analysis of why this was so, with everyone at the meeting taking "joint responsibility" for trying to solve the issue. This process not only keeps conveners and others working on goals accountable and "up to the mark" in what they are meant to do, but also creates a tremendous positive energy, which is vital for the success and resilience of a project. *We believe these processes lie at the heart of a successful project.*

Step 12: Write Guidelines and Set up Educational/ Training Processes

Once people have established themselves in their positions and know what they are doing, it is important for them to write down how to do their job, so that there are guidelines for future people who fill those positions. As alluded to above, this has both an important symbolic function and an important practical function. Symbolically, it is a statement that no one is indispensable, and that the organization is realistically planning for the inevitable fact of personnel turnover and the "empowering" of new people to take on leadership roles. Practically, it means that the painful process undergone by the first person to take on a new role in the organization can be short-circuited in future, and their wisdom and experience can be drawn on for the next person. At the same time the guidelines are seen as being in constant evolution—the next person will learn more about how to do things well, and will modify the guidelines accordingly.

Guidelines also mean that prospective candidates for a position know what is entailed in the job, and also those advertising the position can know exactly what it is they are looking for.

Guidelines are useful for helping to sort out personnel difficulties. Some of the most difficult internal experiences any project is likely to have concern personnel who are not following the philosophy, or who are otherwise not doing the job in a satisfactory way. Often, this is a "personality thing", and can therefore get emotional and confused. We have found that the cleanest way to deal with such difficulties is to have a factual appraisal of the situation by a neutral and trusted adjudicator (such as the Chair of the committee), and this is best done when there are clear guidelines for that person to use about what a job entails.

Guidelines also have an important educational role in a project, and the place of education about the nature and process of a project is a vital matter to consider. For example, whenever new people come into the project, whether staff or "ordinary participants", it is desirable to have available a variety of information and training resources tailored to suit different needs and roles. All of this is geared to ensuring that there is a good understanding of what the project is about and what its processes are.

Step 13: Set up Outcome Evaluation Measures and Processes

This is the final step in the implementation phase. Since outcome evaluation requires major consideration in its own right, it is the topic of the whole of the next chapter, and we leave further discussion until then.

CONCLUSION

In this chapter, we have broken down the People System concept into a series of procedural steps to be considered in setting up a "typical" generic, locality-based community health promotion project that is empowering and under community control. Of course, this is only one kind of project to which PCHP principles and People System methods can be applied, but we hope it gives an illustration of the way in which one can work using this approach. In Chapters 12–14, we cover a number of "real" projects that have used this general approach, and the variety of potential applications is illustrated there. Intrinsic to all these projects is a commitment to outcome evaluation, and we turn to that topic now.

11

THE PEOPLE SYSTEM
Outcome Evaluation

Both PCHP and the People System have evaluation as a key component. Evaluation, as we have said, is more than just a set of methods. Rather, it involves a whole way of looking at an enterprise—one that is constantly addressing two questions: Are we doing this in the best possible way? and Is the whole thing working? This chapter is concerned with the latter of these questions, in the context of People System projects of the type we have been discussing in Chapters 9 and 10.

Conventionally, there is a distinction between "process" and "outcome" evaluation, although these terms seem to mean somewhat different things to different people. In the People System approach, "process evaluation" mainly refers to the review process that we described in the last chapter in the context of the goal-setting and review meeting, which is used primarily for management and organizational purposes to "steer" the "self-optimizing cybernetics system" toward its stated goals, within the context of its philosophy.

However, what we now want to address is the question of "outcome evaluation", which is essentially designed to answer the question: What is the impact of this project? or Is it effective? The world is full of good ideas, with people strongly supporting them. But it is entirely another matter to demonstrate convincingly that these good ideas actually work—that is, that they are better than rival approaches, or better than doing nothing. Some projects may even do harm, or have the opposite effect from what was intended. Ultimately, outcome evaluation is required to vindicate the effort and resources put into any project, and to demonstrate to its community, to those working in it, and to its funders, that it is worth while and effective. Also, hopefully, in a health promotion context, it will be possible to demonstrate that it is having a positive *health* impact.

Before we go into how to do an outcome evaluation, it is worth saying a little more about why such evaluation is desirable.

First, as implied by what we have just said, there is a natural curiosity by the organizers to know if one's project is effective—a bit like "passing an exam".

Second, it is important from the point of view of "accountability", especially as far as the community is concerned. That is, the community is putting a lot into the project. Is it getting something of value out of it? What exactly *is* going on?

Third, outcome evaluations have a management function—they permit one to take stock of the overall enterprise, to determine whether it is broadly on track, and to make overall policy decisions about direction and strategy.

Fourth, to the extent that evaluation outcomes are positive—that they demonstrate positive health effects or other signs of human benefit—then this is powerful information for a variety of public relations and political purposes. Most projects will be concerned with getting financial resources—no project ever has enough money, and often the very survival of a project is at stake. "Data" showing convincingly that a project is effective and having a positive impact provide the basis for a very persuasive argument to those whom one is approaching for support. Such data are also important when a project is seeking political or bureaucratic support for what is being done.

It would be possible to write a whole book on evaluating community development projects, and we do not intend to do that here. Rather, we wish to confine ourselves to evaluation within the context of the People System approach, and to cover that in only enough detail to give you, the reader, an idea of how to proceed. However, we believe that the kind of evaluation approach adopted here is applicable to almost any type of social system endeavour, and can also be applied to individuals and small groups.

For our purposes here, we break the types of relevant evaluation down into the following categories:

- goal attainment
- participation statistics
- surveys
- objective indices
- subjective measures of health and well-being
- satisfaction measures
- qualitative description and research
- quasi-experimental research

At first, this may seem like a somewhat arbitrary list. However, each item is there for a purpose. In most instances of doing an evaluation, one would opt to have several measures to give a rounded picture. Some items are elective, or describe (as in the case of qualitative or quasi-experimental research) a whole research strategy or approach. Others we regard as more or less essential, in particular, goal attainment, participation statistics, subjective measures of health and well-being, and satisfaction measures.

We will now go through these items one by one, explaining the rationale of each, showing how it is done, and describing where we feel it fits into the scheme of things. We also provide examples of the types of summary statements one can make from each source of information.

Goal Attainment

Goal-attainment evaluation answers the questions: Is this project attaining what it sets out to achieve? and Is this project meeting people's needs and wishes? Let us consider the latter first. Is this project meeting people's needs and wishes?

This is a crucial question in the light of the overall thrust of PCHP. That is, in an empowerment context, what drives a community health promotion project is expressed community needs and wishes, systematically ascertained. As outlined in the last chapter, these needs and wishes are assessed through random surveys and other means, then prioritized and translated directly into goals (typically, annual goals). Thus, the assessment of whether people's needs and wishes are being met is a matter of determining (a) whether the goals are an accurate reflection of the expressed needs and wishes, and (b) whether or not the goals have been attained.

The first of these questions, that is whether the goals capture the expressed needs and wishes of the community, is a matter for subjective judgement. However, the public and consultative nature of the goal-setting process goes a long way to ensuring that the goals do represent the true wishes of the community. Furthermore, their continuing existence in the public arena in a visible, written-down form, and their regular use at GSR meetings and other such settings, mean that the goals are constantly under scrutiny. Also, the assessment of whether they have been attained brings up the whole question of the validity of the goals, and how "good" or "relevant" a goal is, so this aspect is, in a way, being indirectly assessed from many points of view a lot of the time.

The second question of whether these goals have actually been attained is, in the People System model, answered through a formal process of review. That is, on the assumption that we are working with annual goals, then once a year, at the time set for all the annual goals to be attained (that is, one year from when they were set), a public meeting is called to present what has happened on each of those goals. As far as possible, the goals have been couched in a language that makes their attainment easy to assess, so that the "goal attainment" is in relatively "objective" terms. For example, a goal of having a childcare facility running for a specified number of sessions a week is readily measurable. The assessment of the attainment of annual goals can use a rating system, an example of which is given for the Birkdale–Beachhaven Community Project in Chapter 12.

Typically, there is not too much trouble assessing the degree of goal attainment. When there are problems, the public nature of the assessment process means that a consensual view is obtained for the rating, and our experience is that this generally tends to be "conservative" (erring on the low rather than the high side). That is, although the goal-attainment ratings are ultimately subjective, they are generally (in our view) fairly accurate and seldom artificially inflated.

This process of rating goal attainment leads to the ability to make evaluative statements about the project in a form such as the following:

In (year), 12 annual goals were set. Of these, nine were fully attained, two mainly attained, and one was abandoned for lack of resources. The goals that were attained related to the following community needs and wishes:

1. To have a place where residents can get together to socialize and plan activities for their community
2. To have a childcare facility that enables parents to leave their children in a high-quality environment, and to give these parents time off to join in community project activities or otherwise have a break from parenting
3. etc.

From this, we conclude that the project was mainly very successful in meeting important expressed needs from the community.

Participation Statistics

Since maximal participation by the community is a goal of PCHP, it is important to determine the penetration of the project into the community of interest, and to find out how many people are involved, and at what level. It will be up to the individual project to determine how to do this, and it is not always straightforward. For example, large and complicated projects may have many different levels of "participation", from leadership roles, through group leaders, to course participants or users of facilities, to different programme members, to those who attend the odd function, to those who may only be indirectly involved, to those who participate in a community activity (such as growing a healthy garden), to school children who participate in project-organized activities, to those who help to raise funds, to . . . well, almost anything.

For evaluation purposes, it is helpful to break participation statistics down into labelled categories, such as those we have just mentioned. But, even at the most basic level, there may be difficulties. For example, it might seem that a project which runs classes of various kinds, and where class lists are kept by group leaders, would provide straightforward data collection. However, a moment's reflection will show that these figures are not necessarily accurate, because the same person may attend several different activities. What is of most importance here is to find out how many *different* people are involved in a project's activities—that is, what *proportion* of the community is involved, and (if possible) who these people are in terms of community representativeness.

On the whole, where large numbers are concerned, and it is not possible to work from detailed records, we feel that "guesstimates" are acceptable, provided there is a commitment to making these err on the conservative side. For example, in one project, we were able to work out a formula from doing a small-scale intensive study for calculating how many people on average went to how many different activities, then we applied this as a "correction" to the overall attendance statistics.

It may also be possible to get the data in more than one way. For example, data gathered through actual participation could be checked against data from a community survey, where an attempt is made to find out how many people take part in project activities. (Surveys also provide the opportunity for demographic breakdowns of the nature of participants.)

Participation data permit us to make statements such as the following:

In (such and such) community, which has a population of 15 000 people, statistics kept by the project showed that it had involved over 10 000 of these people in some shape or form (67% of the total community), of whom 300 were in various leadership or organizational roles, 5000 took direct part in some project activity over a period of time, and the other 5000 had at least one direct contact with a project activity. A survey showed similar rates, and this survey also showed that 95% of the population had heard of the project in the community. A demographic breakdown of survey results showed that all sectors of the community were represented in project activities in approximate proportion to their numbers in the community.

Surveys

We mentioned, just above, one use of a survey in the outcome evaluation area— that of ascertaining or checking participation rates and demographics. Often, with a complicated campaign or project, this may be the only practical way to get such information. A survey is, of course, just a tool, and it can be used to collect many sorts of information. The most valuable form of survey is one that meticulously attempts to get a random sample, so that it is then possible to generalize to the population at large. However, some forms of evaluation might also call for a more qualitative survey approach, using, say, a "snowball" or purposive sampling method. This would be used specifically where in-depth, experiential information is desired. Ideally, most survey-based evaluations would include both quantitative and qualitative approaches.

Objective Indices

What we are referring to here are the kinds of indices one gets from epidemiological research, censuses, medical records, school records, police files, and so on. The task is typically to go to an existing data source, and count what is available there. Or it may be to set up a data collection system to get this sort of information on an ongoing basis. More often than not, these indices tend to be "negative", for example, suicides, family breakdown, child accidents, alcohol-related injury, child abuse cases, unemployment, and so on.

At a superficial level, such data are attractive because they seem to be "scientific". In practice, they are typically fraught with difficulty. For example, existing databases seldom provide exactly the information you want for your evaluation. There may be errors in record-keeping (very common), or the "community" defined by the data-gatherers does not correspond with the boundaries of the community you are interested in, or the classification categories are not quite right, and so on. Also, the available records very often do not catch all the eligible people in a labelled category. For example, using admissions to a psychiatric hospital as an indicator of mental health in a community may be quite misleading. These data may simply reflect the hospital-using habits of one sector of the community and, even then, many in that sector may fall through the cracks. And what would, say, a decrease in the use of something like a psychiatric service mean anyway? A genuine improvement in local mental health? Fewer staff available to see clients? Bad press about the service in the community? The opening of a new and better facility elsewhere? Changed entry or diagnostic criteria by the service? The same kind of critique can be done for almost any "objective" index one might think of. What about increased or decreased cases of sexual abuse? Of suicide? Of police arrests of criminals? Of visits to doctors? Certainly, some data like those available from epidemiological research showing, for example, changed rates in health or disease patterns in a community may be of significance. However, even then, without a properly conducted control study, one may not really know whether it is one's project that has had the impact, or something else.

In short, then, while we certainly do not dismiss the use of so-called "objective" indices, we also feel they should not be oversold. Used in conjunction with other measures, and interpreted responsibly, they have their place. And of course, at their best, for example where such data are derived from a tailored research project with appropriate controls (see "quasi-experimental research"), they are very powerful indeed.

Subjective Measures of Health and Well-being

The simplest way of finding out how well a person is feeling is, of course, to ask him or her. This is typically done for evaluative purposes through the vehicles of questionnaires, rating scales, interviews, and so on, to find out how people judge their own status. Of all measures, they are some of the easiest to collect. But like most of the others, they have both their strengths and weaknesses.

The strengths of subjective measures are several. First, they are easy to get. You simply ask the relevant people to take a few minutes to tell you about themselves, which may or may not involve some sort of "standard" psychological or health test. Second, they go right to the heart of what really matters—how people *experience* their health and their life. Third, they often have a reasonable correlation with more objective measures, such as visits to doctors, blood pressure, time off work, and so on.

The weaknesses of such measures are well known. That is, they *are* subjective, and hence are able to be influenced by all sorts of extraneous matters, such as the desire to please the person doing the evaluation, the desire to put oneself in a good or a bad light for whatever reason, the difficulty of making an accurate judgement about oneself, or even remembering how one was, say, a month or so ago. And although there are often correlations with more objective measures, there are also often quite clear differences, which can be a puzzle.

One other objection to the way subjective measures are sometimes used relates to an issue we raised with regard to "objective" measures. That is, because a change is observed after an intervention or project activity, it does not mean the reported changes have anything significant to do with that project. It may require a controlled study to elucidate these questions, and even then it may be difficult to draw accurate conclusions, mainly because of the difficulty of having truly convincing controls. That is, subjective ratings are very sensitive to all sorts of influences, and if, for example, participants in a research project suspect they have not had the full treatment, or have had some other unusual experience, even if the intention was for them to be "controls", the results may be artificially affected.

One way that we have got around this partially has been by using something we call the "Impact Questionnaire" (Raeburn, 1987). We mention this here, because others may also find it useful.

The Impact Questionnaire was developed to provide a "universal" evaluation measure applicable to any health promotion project. Its aim was to get people to report on their own health and well-being in the following way:

- How do they rate their health and well-being now? (At the end of, or at some other suitable assessment point in, whatever health promotion activity they have been engaged in.)
- How would they have rated their health and well-being when they started this activity?
- If there is a change, would they ascribe that to the health promotion activity?
- Overall, how satisfied were they with the health promotion activity?

As may be seen, this is "universal" for any health promotion activity. It is also subjective, of course. However, what is especially pertinent here is the request for the participant to say whether she or he ascribes any changes to the activity as such. In short, it is asking people to do their own small controlled experiment, in getting them to sort out whether they think the changes are due to the intervention or to other causes. Obviously this is not a perfect solution, but we think it goes some way in the right direction.

Versions of the Impact Questionnaire have been used by a number of different researchers and projects across a variety of cultural settings, and all have found it valuable. (See, for example, the North Shore Community Health Network case study in Chapter 14.) It can be adapted to different settings without an essential loss of meaning. One version (the original one) is shown in Figure 11.1. This was designed to fit in with the scoring categories of a Canadian Social Indicators survey in the early 1980s, so that the "norms" provided by that survey could be used as a base to compare the proportions in the categories found in any subsample. (People should feel free to change these categories to suit their purposes.)

Such a scale, plus other information sources, enables one to make the following kinds of statement:

Following participation in this project, 85% of people said that their state of health had improved either a lot (40%) or somewhat (45%) since first having contact with the project. The majority (90%) ascribed a role to the project in those positive changes, with 60% saying the project had had a lot to do with these changes and 30% a bit to do with them. Eighty per cent said they were able to cope better with life through their contact with the project, and 91% expressed overall satisfaction with the project (67% very satisfied, 24% somewhat satisfied) . . .

IMPACT QUESTIONNAIRE

1. Around the time you first had contact with this project, how would you have described your state of health (compared to other persons your age)?

   1. Excellent   3. Fair
   2. Good   4. Poor

2. Since then, has your state of health improved?

   1. Yes—a lot   3. No—the same
   2. Yes—somewhat   4. No—worse

3. If your health has changed, would you say the project has had anything to do with it?

   1. Yes—a lot   3. No
   2. Yes—a bit   4. Does not apply

4. Around the time you first had contact with this project, how would you have described your overall happiness and well-being?

   1. Very happy   3. Somewhat unhappy
   2. Somewhat happy   4. Very unhappy

5. Since then, have your happiness and well-being improved?

   1. Yes—a lot   3. No—the same
   2. Yes—somewhat   4. No—worse

6. If your happiness and well-being have changed, would you say the project has had anything to do with it?

   1. Yes—a lot   3. No
   2. Yes—a bit   4. Does not apply

7. When you first had contact with the project, were there any particular issues for which you thought the project could be helpful for you personally?

   1. Yes   3. No
   2. No particular ones—just general

8. Did you in fact find the project helpful for these issues (whether particular or general)?

   1. Yes—a lot   3. No—had no effect
   2. Yes—to some extent   4. No—made them worse

9. Overall, would you say that your contact with the project has helped you to cope or manage better in your own life?

   1. Yes—a lot   3. No
   2. Yes—a bit   4. No—had a negative effect

10. Overall, how satisfied have you been with this project?

    1. Very satisfied   3. Somewhat dissatisfied
    2. Somewhat satisfied   4. Very dissatisfied

Figure 11.1:   Impact Questionnaire

Satisfaction Measures

In the example given above, it will be noted that the final statement relates to people's overall satisfaction with the process. This means how much did people like what went on, did they think their participation was worth while, and so on. Such expressions of satisfaction can readily be assessed through self-report questionnaires.

Not only do satisfaction measures relate to overall or global assessments of projects or programmes, but they can be useful to assist with the appraisal of component parts. For example, people can be asked about what they thought of the physical environment of a project, the people running it, the different activities and facilities making up that programme, and so on. This is helpful in working out what to keep, change or eliminate from an under-taking in the future.

Such satisfaction measures can lead to statements of the following kind:

> Of all those taking part in this project, 92% said they were satisfied with their experience with it (60% very satisfied, 32% reasonably satis-fied). When different parts of the project were assessed, 90% expressed satisfaction with those running the activities, 85% said that they had learned a great deal from their participation, and 90% said they liked the format. However, only 25% were satisfied with the premises used, and 75% were bothered by the noisy surroundings. However, 85% said they would recommend another such project to their friends, and 90% said they would like more of the same for themselves.

Qualitative Description and Research

Most of the information described above has been collected in such a way that it can be easily summarized into bite-sized units (often asked in terms of points on a scale or in a multi-choice format), which permits quantitative analysis with the minimum of transformation or coding. While this has obvious advantages, and provides much useful information, it also misses a great deal. In particular, it misses the full richness of people's experience of participating in activities, of empowerment, of a sense of community, of feeling well, and so on. This sort of in-depth, meaningful, experiential infor-mation is what we are referring to as "qualitative" here.

Increasingly, health promotion and social science generally have been discovering the merits of qualitative information, which can never be matched by quantitative data. Such information can be collected relatively informally (though systematically), or it can be analysed by a variety of methods, such as discourse analysis. The disadvantage of such information is that because it is detailed and "dense", it is typically not possible to have large or representative samples, so one loses "coverage" or "generalizability". However, there are emerging methods, such as rapid ethnographic assessment, which are attempts to integrate both the coverage and generality of the quantitative survey approach, with the in-depth and less formal or structured approach of qualitative research.

In short, then, qualitative information is seen as an important element to add "richness", "depth" and "real life" to the other sources of more quantitative evaluative data.

Quasi-experimental Research

In social and behavioural science, the "ideal" for evaluation has usually been the controlled experiment, which permits one to say with some confidence whether changes measured are "significant" (that is, they are not just random changes), whether they can be ascribed to the intervention or to some other cause, and what components of the intervention are the most important ones. In the kind of health promotion setting we are dealing with here, such evaluation is not normally undertaken, except as part of a research project. Also, because of the "naturalistic" nature of the community settings, it is difficult to get the degree of control that is the ideal for controlled research, at least to the degree one can get that control, say, in a laboratory. However, one approach we have used (for an example see Chapter 13) is what is called "quasi-experimental design", which can be seen as a compromise between the tight controls of the laboratory, and the no-controls situation of much programme evaluation in the community.

This is not the place to go into quasi-experimental research methods in detail. But it is worth making some general points.

At the heart of both classical experimental research and quasi-experimental research is the concept of "control". Most people will have heard of the concept of "control groups", and these are relevant here, although not all "control" methods necessarily involve separate groups. (Note: the term "control" in this context has nothing to do with the term "control" as used earlier in this book as a psychological and political phenomenon.) In essence, the idea of control in a research setting is to guard against the error implicit in the expression, *post hoc, ergo propter hoc*—that is, just because some change follows some event, it has not necessarily been caused by that event. In general, the tighter the controls in an experiment, the more we are in a position to make statements about what is going on with the minimum likelihood of error.

In psychology, and most other social science, the ideal experimental design involving groups of people either inside or outside the laboratory is called the "random groups design". Here, people are allocated to experimental and control groups (the simplest configuration being where one group ("experimental") gets an intervention and the other ("control") does not on a random basis, perhaps by the toss of a coin or some other method. What this does is attempt to equalize the characteristics of the people in the two groups, and most standard statistical methods are designed on the assumption that the people in the various groups being compared are from "the same population" (to use the statistical jargon).

In most community development research, it is difficult to get random allocation to groups. We have tried on a number of occasions to do so, and have had to give up. Instead, one can use "quasi-experimental" designs. Quasi-experimental designs attempt to approximate classical experimental conditions as much as possible, but do not have the fundamental requirement of random allocation. For example, one quasi-experimental design we commonly use is that involving "waiting-list controls". People wanting to take part in an activity that is being studied for research purposes are enrolled as participants in the order they contact the organizers, until the roll is full. This is called the "study group". Any further people are then put on to a waiting list until the activity can be run again, but while they are waiting they undergo the same assessment procedures at the same time as their colleagues who got into the study group. These waiting-list people are called the "control" or "comparison group". This is quite an effective design because the controls are people who are similarly motivated to those in the experimental group, an important variable in most health promotion research. However, the fact that the controls were slower off the mark to enrol than those who came first may say something about them as people, which could affect the final outcome—a problem that at least theoretically is neutralized with random allocation. Also, the fact of having to wait, and especially perhaps missing the crucial time of deciding to (say) change a lifestyle habit, means that waiting-list controls are far from being "the same" as the study group.

There are a number of quasi-experimental designs, all of which are aimed at getting the maximum control under difficult circumstances. As far as the PCHP researcher is concerned, any such projects would be designed, of course, in full partnership with the community of interest. Often, there may have to be compromises on both sides to meet the requirements both of the research and of not interfering with the activities and life of the people concerned to any great degree. And, here, one has to make a distinction between "evaluation" of the type we have been talking about for most of this chapter, and "research", which is a "deeper" enterprise. Basically, with evaluation, we just want to know if something is working. In "research", we also want to know how and why it is working. In this regard, the use of such an approach is more in the realm of research than straight evaluation. Research will tell you such things as (a) whether such a project is doing better than having nothing at all, (b) whether some options are better than other options, (c) whether there is a real effect of the project over and above a "placebo" or "general mobilization" impact, (d) whether this community with a project is doing better than another community without such a project, and (e) whether this project is performing better or worse than a comparable one elsewhere.

Quasi-experimental designs do not necessarily exhaust the types of controlled research possibilities in a community development setting. Sometimes full experimental trials may be possible. Also, adaptations of single-subject control designs and time-series types of designs may also be applicable.

SUMMARY STATEMENT OF AN EVALUATION

To give you a "flavour" of the sort of summary statements possible from our approach to evaluation, we include a hypothetical example here. Although slightly idealized, it is similar to those we have actually produced in various projects (see Chapters 12–14). Such statements can be used when dealing with politicians or funding bodies.

This project was aimed at improving the health and well-being of the people of the (such and such) community through building community spirit, meeting important goals ascertained from the community, and getting maximal participation in project activities. To do this, annual goals were set, to cover activities deemed desirable and important by the community. The project has now been running for five years, and in the last year of operation, 12 annual goals were set. Of these 12 goals, 11 were fully attained and one was partly attained. The activities generated by these goals involved two-thirds of the community of all ages and backgrounds at a variety of levels. Of these people, 85% reported feeling healthier and happier after having had a contact with the project, and 90% ascribed these improvements to their involvement in the project. Also, 92% felt satisfied or very satisfied with their experience with the project. A random survey also found that residents felt that community spirit had increased during the existence of the project, and the levels of participation and satisfaction were also confirmed by this survey. Of note also is that all sectors of the community were equally involved in project activities, although

continues

— *continued* —

there was a preponderance of women over men (70% were women). Statistics obtained from the police and other agencies showed that juvenile crime rates have dropped by 40% since the beginning of the project, and house sales have also dropped, suggesting that people wanted to stay in this community rather than move out. Data from schools and health services showed that numbers of teenage suicides have fallen significantly from previous "epidemic" levels, and Social Welfare reported less family breakdown and violence. A quasi-experimental research study comparing this community with two other communities of similar demography and characteristics showed that all measurable changes were significantly positive compared with indices for the other communities, which either stayed the same or slightly deteriorated over the same period of time. Qualitative studies confirmed the overall impression of a favourable and health-promoting response to the project, and many said that it was the best thing that had ever happened to the community.

CONCLUSION

This chapter, and Chapters 9 and 10, were aimed at providing practical guidelines, using the People System, for setting up and evaluating PCHP projects of a community-development type. This is, however, only one type of application of this general approach, and in the next three chapters we will see a number of variations on this theme, as we cover a number of real-life cases. As we said before, the People System approach is not intended to provide a hard and fast set of rules—it is simply an orderly, and indeed common-sense, approach, which works well for enterprises of this nature, and which can be adapted and reshaped as required. Likewise, the outcome evaluation component we considered in this chapter can be adapted to the requirements and resources of a given situation.

One important virtue of this whole approach, with regard both to organization and to evaluation, is that it *does* make sense to the ordinary person. Although sophisticated and capable of producing data of an "academic" standard, these ways of going about things make sense to anyone, and are readily understood in their intent and operation. From this point of view, they are very suitable for community undertakings, where empowerment and community control are central issues. That is, these processes can be understood and owned by the people themselves, and adapted by them, since they know what the principles are. This is very important, since so much of what seems to spoil the relationship between professional and community is the professional seeming to be the possessor of "esoteric" or "special" knowledge to which the "common herd" is denied access. The People System approach puts the professional's powerful tools into the hands of the people themselves.

In applying the People System, what counts is not the slavish application of a neat organizational procedure, but an overall approach that is true to the values of positively experienced health, empowerment, community development, community control, cultural appropriateness, and so on, which are at the heart of PCHP. In the chapters that follow, we hope this diversity and flexibility of application is illustrated.

12

CASE STUDIES I
Community Push and the Birkdale–Beachhaven Community Project

In this and the next two chapters, we look at projects that exemplify the development and application of the PCHP philosophy, and how the People System approach can be used to operationalize this in a practical way.

Here, it should be noted that the terms PCHP and People System are to some extent used interchangeably. The "how to do it" dimension, which is what this part of the book is about, is in terms of the People System. But the underlying value system and philosophy is PCHP.

In what follows, then, the discussion is mainly in terms of the People System, but some of the examples are followed by an analysis in terms of PCHP, to show how PCHP principles are being observed in a number of quite divergent settings and enterprises.

The examples that follow are all from a New Zealand setting. This is because, of the two authors, John Raeburn has been the principal user of this approach, and these examples are all projects he has personally been involved with. The People System (not always called by that name) was an approach he and others developed as a result of attempting to take a systematic and evaluative approach to setting up community health promotion projects with a PCHP type of philosophy.

The approach now called the "People System" evolved from a number of research projects spanning more than 20 years. The projects covered in Chapters 12–14 by no means exhaust the possible examples. Rather, they have been chosen to illustrate a diversity of applications, and also to illustrate the continuing evolution of such an approach. Although to some this approach may seem overly prescriptive and "organized", we hope the examples given here will show that it is actually very flexible, and considerable liberties can be taken with it, so long as the core principles are observed.

In this chapter, two of the earliest examples of the use of a PCHP/People System approach are given, covering the period 1972–1980. In Chapter 13, we present the Superhealth programmes, involving lifestyle-oriented health promotion in a community setting, and covering the period approximately from 1975 to 1989. Then, in Chapter 14, we look at two more recent cases, one of which is still in a development phase, covering the period from 1983 to the present. As these dates suggest, these projects are inevitably long-term undertakings, requiring a great deal of slow development time. However, this groundwork pays off, if by no other criterion than longevity—many of these projects still exist in some form today.

The aim is to give these examples not so much as conventional research reports, such as one would find in the academic literature (even though most have been written up and published that way), but as more of a lived experience. Unfortunately, space does not permit a lot of detail of the day-to-day processes of these projects, which is where the life of them really is, but we hope something of their "feel" comes through. One is not looking for "scientific objectivity" under these circumstances, although we do present some formally derived research data. (If readers want more of the research side than is given here, they will need to look up the relevant references, which are given in the text.)

The case studies begin with an early 1970s project called "Community Push". As will be seen, this was not a health promotion project or even a community-based project, but a rehabilitation programme located in a psychiatric ward. But it represents an early attempt at applying PCHP-type principles, which in turn had been inspired by the American "community mental health movement" of the 1960s, and so had a strong community flavour (e.g. see Thackeray et al., 1979). Many of the basics of the People System were established in this project. Then we proceed to the major section of this chapter, which concerns a concept called the "community house" as first developed in the Birkdale–Beachhaven Community Project.

In Chapter 13, we describe a series of healthy lifestyle programmes called "Superhealth", which grew out of the community house projects. While these are not community development programmes as such, they are inspired by PCHP principles, and they are unquestionably community-based health promotion, as that term was understood in those days before the Ottawa Charter.

In Chapter 14, the first of the two cases looks at something called an "Empowering Resource Centre", as embodied in the North Shore Community Health Network. This concerns the area of "mental health promotion", and has a regional rather than a locality perspective. The second case in Chapter 14, and the final one we cover, is a new project, still in a developmental phase at the time of writing this book, called the "Other Way Project". It represents a contemporary approach to generic locality-based community development with a health promotion agenda.

So, now to the first example, which is probably best seen as a forerunner to the PCHP/People Systems approach—a psychiatric ward-based rehabilitation programme called "Community Push".

THE COMMUNITY PUSH PROGRAMME (1972–1973)

This project was initiated in 1972 in a busy, short-stay psychiatric ward located on the tenth floor of Auckland Hospital. The prevailing treatment ethos was then conventional chemotherapy and ECT, combined with psychotherapeutic groups of a psychodynamic and "encounter group" nature. Apart from the contribution of an active social work team, there was little orientation of the ward programmes to the community, and little attention was given to practical living skills.

Community Push started as an attempt to initiate a comprehensive evaluation programme on the ward, to be conducted under the auspices of the University of Auckland's Department of Psychiatry. To do this, it was decided to set up an entirely new programme, which would "model" how evaluation could be done.

Although the original impetus for the project was to establish an evaluation programme, increasingly it changed to being an experiment in how to set up a community-oriented rehabilitation programme for patients who had not responded to the regular ward treatments being offered. Over the 15 months the programme was in existence, 76 patients went through Community Push. (Note: the term "patient" was in common use in psychiatric services at that time, so we continue that usage here.)

The community mental health and allied evaluative literature of that period suggested that the optimal way to set about evaluation in a context like this was through the use of goals. Also, it was clear that "needs assessment", that is allowing patients to articulate their own needs and wishes ascertained in a systematic way, was desirable. The Community Push "system" was set up with its overall goal being "to facilitate successful functioning in the community". The overall philosophy was one of enabling the patient to set his or her own agenda, and then using a wide variety of volunteers and community resources to meet personal goals determined by the patient to be necessary for successful functioning in the community.

The process consisted of the following steps: (1) An assessment interview (about one hour) was done, where the interviewer and patient jointly went though the main areas of community functioning, then drew up a list of needs and prioritized these. (2) Concrete goals with deadlines were specified and written down from these prioritized needs. Each goal was given a rating

of A, B or C, on a scale of A = essential for the person's successful
functioning in the community; B = highly desirable to achieve; C = good to
attend to if there is time. The goal was then allocated a staff or other resource
person who would assist the patient to achieve it. In addition, each patient
had a "mentor", a staff person who coordinated that patient's programme of
goals, and who acted as a general counsellor and friend. (3) Action on goals
was taken by engaging in practical matters such as learning social skills,
finding accommodation, getting a job, making new friends, and so on. In
general, the emphasis was on the development of "strengths" (new skills,
etc.) and on people taking their own action, with the facilitation and back-up
of others. For some of the goals, resources were already available on the
ward or in the community. For others, new activities had to be set up. In
addition, each patient belonged to a group of six to eight people, which
existed for support, encouragement on achieving goals, and general matters.
This group also formed the basis of a subsequent follow-up group. (4)
Weekly goal-review sessions were held in which staff monitored progress
on all goals for all patients in the programme. (5) Voluntary follow-up
groups continued for patients until they had completed their goals. (6) An
outcome evaluation summary was done at 18 months, which was when the
programme was forced to finish.

One feature of this project was the extensive use of volunteers. In general,
the aim was to find volunteers who lived reasonably close to the patient,
who could assist with one or more goals. By the time the programme ended,
more than 80 volunteers were participating.

The outcome evaluation at 18 months showed the following:

> The principal diagnoses of the 76 patients [who entered the programme] were
> neurosis (29%), psychosis (23%), and personality disorder (21%). Most had
> received previous psychiatric treatment . . . Of the 76 patients, only 54 com-
> pleted their CP programmes. Of the other 22, 4 withdrew voluntarily and 18
> were discharged by their doctors for a variety of reasons unconnected with CP.
> Of the 54 staying in the programme, 42 (78%) were a "total success" in terms of
> goal-attainment (i.e. they successfully completed all their goals) . . .
>
> The number of goals set per patient ranged from one to seven, with an
> average of four. For the 76 patients entering the programme, there was a total
> of 309 goals set and 182 (59%) attained.
>
> . . . For the 76 patients entering the programme the types of goals set were
> (in order): domestic (23%), social relationships (20%), spare time (20%), occupa-
> tional (15%), medical and psychiatric (9%), finance and business (6%) and
> personal philosophy (6%). The majority of the 309 goals (70%) were considered
> important enough to be given an "A" priority rating which said: "It is essential
> to deal with this goal if the patient is to function in the community". (Raeburn,
> 1976, pp. 307–308)

Unfortunately, resources and the sudden demise of the programme did
not permit a follow-up study.

In terms of PCHP principles, Community Push can be assessed as follows:

1. People-centredness

Community Push was grounded in the practical everyday community experience of ordinary people, rather than being "esoteric" or special, as seemed to be the case for much of the psychotherapy that was taking place on the ward.

2. Empowerment

The term "empowerment" was not in currency when Community Push was developed, but it is clear that a number of empowerment dimensions were operative here. First, a good deal of the control of what was going on was by the patient, and also by the groups to which the patient belonged. Second, most of the activities were geared towards the development of strengths, and establishing a normal, independent life in the community, rather than dependency on a therapist or agency.

3. Organizational and Community Development

Overall, the Community Push programme was based broadly on what could be called an organizational development model, with its goals, reviews, evaluation systems, etc. However, it was not really a community development exercise as such.

4. Participation

The climate of Community Push was a participatory one. Patients were seen as "real people" who were participating in the management of their own lives and programmes, rather than having the professionals or institution do everything for them.

5. Life Quality

A deliberate effort was made in Community Push to have as its domain the whole of a person's life, and to try to see that life as a totality. Also, the goals were all seen as *positive* matters—the translation of negativities (problems, needs) into positive, constructive, satisfying action.

6. Evaluation

It will be remembered that evaluation was the main trigger for Community Push. An evaluation "agenda" was at the basis of the goal-oriented approach, of the needs assessments, of the reviews, of the desire to keep optimizing what was going on, and of the outcome information that was given above.

Conclusion

The Community Push programme was neither a health promotion project nor a community development project as these things are usually understood. Yet it can be seen that it had elements of these aspects in it, and in particular its emphasis on quality of life and positive goals made it almost a health promotion programme rather than a treatment programme.

THE BIRKDALE–BEACHHAVEN COMMUNITY PROJECT (1973–1980)

The cessation of the Community Push programme led to a search in the community for a location to do something similar, but with a community base rather than a hospital one. Eventually, two adjoining suburban areas on the North Shore of Auckland, Birkdale and Beachhaven, were chosen as the place to try to "do something". These two communities were at that time (1973) two of the fastest growing new suburban areas in New Zealand. The development that had taken place had been haphazard, with a variety of types of housing ranging from state rental areas, catering for those on social welfare benefits and low incomes, to some conspicuously affluent housing by the sea. A demographic breakdown revealed that the area represented a cross-section of socio-economic groups in much the same proportions as in the overall population, with most in the low to low-middle income bracket.

Because of the preponderance of new housing, there were many young families with children, often preschoolers. Indeed, about half the total population of the 14 000 people comprising Birkdale and Beachhaven were children of school age or younger.

Birkdale and Beachhaven were served by five schools, three primary, one intermediate and one high school. The impetus to "do something" came from the schools, and from social service and health personnel who were aware of the challenges facing a new community of this type, with its many children and isolated families. In particular, there was concern about the almost complete absence of accessible social services in the area.

The school principals, together with social workers, public health nurses, and other educational and social service personnel, had been meeting regularly to see how they could avert what they characterized as a "social volcano". In particular, they were concerned about the obvious educational disadvantage of a number of the school entrants, the rates of family breakdown, the high juvenile crime rate, and the level of psychological and social disturbance among the children they were seeing at the schools. It was also clear that the community was lacking in recreational facilities for all ages, and there was generally a lack of community spirit, identity and co-hesiveness. This group felt strongly that rather than single out the "problem people" in the community, the aim should be to involve the "whole community", with the aim of getting as many people as possible participating in whatever was done. Therefore, it was decided to adopt an entirely positive way of operating, so that everyone in the community would feel attracted to participate without fear of being labelled negatively by their neighbours.

A second value espoused by this group was to do with "quality of life" as an overall goal. That is, it was felt that action should not be directed at patching up problems, but rather to increase community spirit and the well-being of the whole community.

A third important value was a commitment to needs assessment. That is, it was strongly felt that the agendas for action should be set by the community itself.

It would take a whole book to describe the development of the Birkdale–Beachhaven Community Project (BBCP) over the next seven years, the period it was a "research project". (At the time of writing, the BBCP is still flourishing, and in 1995 it had a celebration of its 20th birthday with events that lasted five days!)

The first meetings to discuss the project were in 1973. By the end of 1974, three things had happened. One was a consensus on how to proceed, and what values would be the guiding principles. Second, it had been decided that there should be a small-scale, friendly, house-based centre for the project. This was obtained, and in time became to be called simply "The House". Third, it was decided to use as "consultants" the "experts" from the university who had joined this group. These people would not run the project, but would nevertheless be allowed to have an important role in seeing it through its inception and organizational aspects, and also would be allowed to treat it as "research".

The first major action was a needs-assessment survey that used a stratified random sample of 100 households, and revealed a clear set of community priorities. The needs-assessment process also included key person interviews, community meetings and a variety of other inputs that confirmed and clarified these priorities. Then a public goal-setting exercise ("public" in the sense that it was widely advertised, and ran over several weeks in various locations) translated these priorities into an initial set of 14 annual goals, to be fulfilled by 1 September 1976.

The initial survey was divided into two main domains of social/recreational and social services. The needs that emerged reflected very much the "young family" nature of the community, with priorities in the areas of preschool facilities, activities and social interaction opportunities for young parents (especially mothers), teenagers, after-school programmes for school children, and the elderly. These need areas were translated into 14 projects grouped into four more general areas: "Good Facilities and Services for All Ages" (e.g. preschool facilities, after-school programmes, teenage facilities, adult activities, over-50s survey), "Development of People's Own Strengths" (e.g. weight control, personal development, communication), "Friendly Relationships between People" (e.g. street-level gatherings), and "Administrative" (e.g. fund-raising, setting up incorporated society). These kinds of projects developed for several years, and reached a height around 1980. Table 12.1 shows what the annual goals looked like in 1980, together with the judged attainment of these goals at the review meeting held in November 1980.

In 1975, an important step was the forming of an incorporated society to run the project. This had the name The Birkdale–Beachhaven Community Project Inc., and its constitutional objects give a good overview of what was intended at that time:

(a) To promote the well-being of the Community encompassed by the areas usually known as Birkdale and Beachhaven (hereinafter called "the community").

(b) To promote opportunities for people in the community to lead effective and satisfying lives by fostering and aiding learning in the individual, and by encouraging and where possible implementing appropriate changes in the physical or social environment.

(c) To promote and protect the principle of community involvement and participation in activities and services relating to the well-being of the community and to ensure that channels are available for such participation.

(d) To encourage the expression and identification of individual, family and community needs, with a view to implementing action appropriate to dealing with these needs.

(e) To facilitate the use of existing social services by ensuring that services are readily accessible to the user, and by providing a venue for the coordination of a wide variety of services.

(f) To promote the principle that those involved in providing services should be accountable for their actions to the community as a whole, as well as to their parent organizations.

(g) To facilitate the development of new services designed to meet those individual, family and community needs not already met by existing services.

(h) To assign priority to the prevention of serious problems through early intervention, community education, and the improvement of community facilities.

(i) To promote the objective evaluation of the process and outcome of services operating in the community.

(j) To encourage services to remain flexible and open to change according to need and to the directions indicated by new information and evaluative data.

(k) To promote research related to the interests of the community.

Table 12.1: Annual goals for 1980

Goals to be attained by November 1980[1]	Judged attainment[2]
1. *Birkdale and Beachhaven Community Houses:* To have continued to run the Birkdale and Beachhaven Community Houses at least at the existing level, which includes having had a full House Roster at both Houses, and Adult Activities and Living Skills at least at 1979 levels. (M)	B
2. *Birkdale and Beachhaven Community Crèches:* To have continued to run at least four sessions at Birkdale Crèche and three sessions at the Beachhaven Crèche up to BBCP standards (i.e. at least one crèche supervisor per session; at least three volunteer helpers per session; support for all crèche staff; equipment and materials to Dept of Education specification) and to have explored and evaluated the number of sessions needed at each crèche. (M & E)	B
3. *Human Development:* To have continued the Human Development Programme at Birkdale Crèche with involvement of fourth form Family Life students at least at the 1979 level, which includes having one particular person who takes responsibility for college students during sessions, apart from the Supervisor or Supervisors, and who is funded by the Dept of Education. (M)	A
4. *Highbury Community Development:* To have established Highbury House and associated crèche sessions, which includes having a full House Roster, Adult Activities and Living Skills available; having obtained a provisional licence from the Dept of Social Welfare to run crèche sessions at Highbury House and to have a minimum of two crèche sessions per week running to BBCP standards. (N)	B
5. *Community Liaison:* To have taken action on the following areas having arisen from needs assessment: small, local neighbourhood playing areas for young children; a public swimming pool in the Birkdale–Beachhaven area; the establishment of trading bank facilities at Beachhaven. (N)	A
6. *School-age Children:* To have further investigated the area of after-school custodial care for primary school aged children, and to have had a report presented to the Project. (E)	A
7. *Teenage Area:* To have investigated the teenage needs area, with a view to positive action and to have had a report presented to the Project. (E)	A
8. *Community Workshop:* To have further investigated resources and facilities for a Community Workshop and to have had a report presented to the Project. (E)	E
9. *Living Skills:* *Parenting:* To have continued to provide educational opportunities for parents by modelling at crèche, and discussion groups and classes for parents of children of all ages. (M)	C

(continues overleaf)

Table 12.1 *(continued)*

Goals to be attained by November 1980[1]	Judged attainment[2]
To have explored the possibility of Parent Groups being run by trained volunteers with professional support. (E)	A
Waistline: To have continued Waistline at least at the 1979 level, and to have implemented whatever maintenance system has been decided on. (EX)	A
Communication Skills: To have continued to run Communication Skills at least at the 1979 level. (M)	A
Unstress: To have evaluated the pilot stages of Unstress, and to have decided on future direction. (N)	A
Self-relaxation: To have explored the need for continuing Self-relaxation classes, and to have continued or discontinued them accordingly. (E)	E
10. *Social Services:* To have continued to run the Social Services group in response to community need. (M)	B
11. *Evaluation and Needs Assessment:* To have maintained needs assessment and evaluation procedures at the 1979 level, and to investigate ways of measuring the social impact of the Project on the community. (M)	A
12. *Constitution and Committee:* To have rewritten and brought up to date the BBCP constitution to a standard acceptable to the Project. This includes a review of the function and role of the committee. (N)	C
13. *Public Relations and Publicity:* To have established a working Public Relations and Publicity group for the BBCP which will include having prepared a handbook giving information of use to prospective and existing committee members, and to the general public. (N)	C
14. *Project Coordination:* To have employed two persons for Project coordination for 20 hours per week per person, which will have included coordination and support of every area listed from 1 to 14 in these proposed Annual Goals. (N)	B
15. *Project Crèche Staff:* To have employed six persons to run all crèche sessions, provide support for parents and take responsibility for community liaison as per Annual Goals. (N)	A

[1] Goals are classified as New (N), Maintenance (M), Exploratory (E) and Expansion (EX), depending on their age and status. That is, after five years, many of the goals were left-overs from previous years (and perhaps were being expanded), others were new, and others were being explored in a needs-assessment or trial fashion.

[2] Judged attainment of these goals at the review meeting held in November 1980: A = fully achieved, B = mostly achieved, C = half achieved, D = somewhat achieved, E = nothing achieved.

The society had the power to employ people, and in 1975 a project coordinator was appointed and paid for 20 hours a week. Because of the importance ascribed to preschool activities, two crèche supervisors (trained preschool workers) were also paid for a few hours a week to run the preschool project, called the "Community Crèche". Later, other people were also employed in a variety of posts, but with a rule that no one was paid for more than 20 hours, to prevent the tendency for one or more persons to take over control.

The project continued to expand for several years. In 1976, a second community house opened (Beachhaven House) as part of the project, and, in 1978, the project expanded to an adjoining community (total population 20 000), added another house, and changed its name to the "Birkenhead Community Project". (It later returned to being just two houses, and reverted to its original name of BBCP.)

So what sort of impact did the project have? There was never a full-scale funded research project associated with the evaluation aspect of the BBCP, and the outcome evaluative information is therefore somewhat piecemeal. Using the headings for outcome evaluation in Chapter 11, the following seemed to have been the impact in the period 1975–1980, when the research was active.

1. Goal Attainment

Annual goals were set each year, and were reviewed at the end of that year. We do not have the records for each year, but we know that at the end of the first year of operation, "15 of 17 projects had fully attained their goals" (Raeburn and Seymour, 1979). The data shown in Table 12.1 for 1980 are probably a reasonable indication of the level of goal attainment later in the project.

2. Participation Statistics

Over the six years being considered here, participation statistics were calculated as follows, with the percentage of the population involved being given in parentheses (note that between 1978, when the third community house opened, and 1980, the population base went from 14 000 to 20 000).

1975:   400 (3% of 14 000)
1976:   2000 (14% of 14 000)
1977:   4000 (28% of 14 000)
1978:   5000 (35% of 14 000 or 25% of 20 000)
1979:   no data
1980:   8000–10 000 (60–70% of 14 000 or 40–50% of 20 000)

In addition, the numbers of people in leadership roles (paid staff, preschool workers, activity group leaders, committee members, etc.) were calculated, and by 1980 had reached approximately 300.

3. Surveys

Over the evaluative period under consideration here, two major community surveys were done, one in 1975 and one in 1978. The 1978 survey followed approximately the same format as was used in 1975, although some changes were made to accommodate the evolving nature of the project, and new issues that might have come up. By 1978, it was clear that the project had had a major impact on the community and, in general, facilities and services were better, and people were less preoccupied with early childhood and "survival" matters. In 1978 it was evident that interests had moved primarily to adult personal development.

The 1978 survey was undertaken when the project was being expanded to include the whole of Birkenhead City, with a population of about 20 000 people, and so the sample is based on this total population. The 1978 survey showed that about 18% of Birkenhead residents were involved in the project (about 25% of Birkdale–Beachhaven). These figures are less than the 1978 participation statistics given above, which came out of a "guesstimate" exercise, and it may be safer to accept the survey results as more accurate. However, the criteria for "participation" could well have been different as well. Regardless, it is safe to say that substantial numbers of people were involved. Of those who were involved, the 1978 survey showed that 77% of these had found their contact with the project "very satisfactory" or "satisfactory". The same survey showed that 90% of adult residents said that they liked living in that community, and 80% said that they got on well with their neighbours.

It is worth noting that, in 1982, an independent newspaper survey found Birkenhead, along with one other suburb, to be the best-liked community in which to live in Auckland, a far cry from its status 10 years earlier (*Auckland Star*, 1982).

4. Objective Indices

No systematic attempt was made to gather the kinds of statistics that would be relevant here (suicide rates, family breakdown rates, school drop-outs, etc.). Therefore, the evidence in this area is anecdotal. Two examples of this follow. First, the North Shore police noted that, during the period we are talking about, the juvenile crime rate in Birkdale–Beachhaven went from being the highest in their district to the lowest, and they ascribed this directly to the presence of the project. Second, the high-school principal reported a fall in teenage pregnancies at the school, which he attributed directly to the school's involvement in the BBCP's preschool programme.

5. Subjective Measures of Health and Well-being

No systematic attempt was made to obtain these measures for the project as a whole. However, some of the subprojects, especially those in the health and personal development area, asked evaluative questions about health and well-being. In general, they showed that these programmes had a marked impact on people's reported health and well-being, and we cover these data in more detail when we look at the Superhealth programmes in Chapter 13.

6. Satisfaction Measures

In general, the data for satisfaction measures come from the surveys, on which we have already reported. For example, we noted above that 77% of those who had had some contact with the project in 1978 reported satisfaction with that contact.

7. Qualitative Description and Research

No formal qualitative research was undertaken with regard to this project. However, there are a number of sources of "qualitative" information that add to the general picture of how the project operated and what impact it had. For example, it could be argued that the growth and survival of such a project is an important indicator in its own right.

Also, the project has had a considerable national impact. The concept of the "community house" was adopted by many other communities throughout New Zealand, many explicitly modelled on the BBCP. At present, there are at least 200–300 such community houses throughout the country.

There is also evidence of a more anecdotal nature about the success of the project in the period 1975–1980. For example, in 1979, under the headline " 'Best project in NZ' gets $5500", the local newspaper reported:

> A Ministry of Recreation and Sport grant of $5500 has been made to the Birkdale–Beachhaven Community Project . . . The grant was announced this week by Birkenhead MP and Minister of Justice Mr Jim McLay. "As a strong supporter of the project since its inception, I am aware of the scope of its programme and the spirit it has engendered in the community", said Mr McLay . . . Mr McLay says he is proud to be associated with the project which he considers is the best community project operating in the country and an

excellent model for others to work from. (*North Shore Times Advertizer*, 24 May 1979)

In the brochure put out in 1995 for the BBCP's 20th-anniversary celebrations, Ann Hartley, the original project coordinator during the 1975–1980 period (and who subsequently went on to be a prominent local government politician and mayor), said the following:

> Many people who shared dreams and visions in 1975 when we established Birkdale Community Project I'm sure would feel 20 years later those dreams had come true. The Community Houses have been a resounding success. This success has spread right throughout New Zealand where many communities have adopted the Community House model.
>
> Birkdale House started because a group of people believed in the concept of people working together to meet their own needs. In 1975 when people were asked (and being asked rather than told was a new concept too) what they wanted to see happen in their community, it was found that one of the greatest needs was for assistance for people with pre-schoolers, and I believe that giving a strong emphasis to this area is why the Community Houses have been successful . . .
>
> The Community is very different from 20 years ago. However, I believe that the things we do together, what we give to one another through our communities, is what our spiritual being is all about. A sense of belonging is just as important as it ever was. In giving we always receive more, and my hope is that the Community Houses will go from strength to strength and continue to be the focus that they are in 1995.

8. Quasi-experimental and Other Controlled Research

There was no overall quasi-experimental or controlled study associated with the whole project. However, as will be seen in Chapter 13, a quasi-experimental approach was taken to the evaluation of the lifestyle programmes associated with this project.

Conclusion

To sum up, we have seen that the Birkdale–Beachhaven Community Project is a comprehensive community development project in a modern suburban setting, where the overall aim was that of increasing the well-being of as many people as possible in the community—and, by implication, their health and quality of life. Although we do not have definitive data to demonstrate these things, we can conclude that the project did have a major participatory impact on the community, that most people were positive about it, and many expressed considerable satisfaction with their community in a way that was not evident before the project started. To the extent that the project did attain its objectives, we believe this can largely be ascribed to its empowerment and community-building philosophy—one where all activities were seen in the context of building people's strengths, and the strengths of the community as a whole. At the heart of this was the attempt to ascertain what the community really wanted, and to base all action on this information.

13

CASE STUDIES II

Superhealth

In the community house project described in Chapter 12, "health promotion" was seen as a broad quality of life matter, associated with living in a strong, supportive community and participating in empowering and beneficial activities. However, within the context of that project were a number of activities that were more classically of a health promotion variety, at least as that term was understood in the 1970s and early 1980s.

As was mentioned in Chapter 12, the surveys showed a considerable amount of community interest in what might be called "personal development" activities, and by the second survey these became the dominant interest. This interest was also found in other communities where similar community house surveys were done. For example, Table 13.1 shows the results obtained when interest in lifestyle and personal development activities was surveyed in three communities, two in Auckland (Birkenhead and Devonport), and one in a rural town, whose population was 50% Maori (Kawakawa) (Raeburn, 1985).

As can be seen, in all three communities, two-thirds or more (68.5–90.0%) of the populations surveyed were interested in lifestyle and personal development activities, and in each case the priorities were for fitness, weight control and stress management. As a result of this kind of information, it was decided to develop, as a research project, "empowering resources" that could be used and owned by community people for

One of the dedications at the beginning of this book is to Joan Atkinson, who participated in the BBCP as a community person in the early years, and then became increasingly interested in the lifestyle programmes. Joan subsequently worked as a principal developer of the Superhealth programmes, over a period of more than 10 years. Her beautiful nature, her talent, her sensitivity, her creativity, and her wonderful manner with people at all levels were incomparable. It is a tragic irony that not long after she finished this work, she died of cancer, still a young woman. She is someone many of us will always remember with the greatest affection.

Table 13.1: Positive responses to questionnaires surveying interest in lifestyle and personal development activities in three communities, ranked in order of priority

Priority	Birkenhead (Nyes = 183 (68.5%); Ntot = 267)			Devonport (Nyes = 106 (70.7%); Ntot = 150)			Kawakawa (Nyes = 45 (90.0%); Ntot = 50)		
		n	%		n	%		n	%
1	Fitness	84	31.5	Fitness	42	28.0	Fitness	21	42
2	Weight	69	25.8	Weight	24	16.0	Stress/tension	16	32
3	Stress/tension	50	18.7	Stress/tension	22	14.7	Weight	15	30
4	Communication	40	15.0	Smoking	17	11.3	Communication	14	28
5	Smoking	36	13.5	Communication	16	10.7	Budgeting	14	28
6	Fear/depression	30	11.2	Health promotion	14	9.3	Health promotion	12	24
7	Confidence	28	10.5	Drug education	13	8.7	Confidence	9	18
8				Alternative medicine	11	7.3	Drug education	9	18
9				Confidence	9	6.0	Smoking	7	14
10				Fear/depression	9	6.0	Assertion	7	14
11				Budgeting	5	4.7	Alcohol education	5	10
12				Alcohol education	2	1.3	Depression/fears	5	10
13				Marriage enhancement	2	1.3	Alternative medicine	4	8
14				Assertion	2	1.3	Marriage preparation	4	8
15				Marriage preparation	1	0.7	Marriage enhancement	4	8

Nyes = number replying to any choice other than "Not interested"; Ntot = total sample surveyed; rankings are of items other than "Not interested", "Interested but not specific", and "Other". Note that the Birkenhead list is shorter because there were fewer choices offered in that survey. Reproduced by permission of NZ Medical Association from Raeburn (1985).

themselves, but which incorporated the latest approaches to health and behaviour change in these various areas. The kinds of setting envisaged for these activities were small groups (up to nine people) in community houses, although they could potentially be used anywhere. The agenda was both behavioural and health change in the area of interest, plus a "community-building" aspect, aimed at developing local support and friendship and also as a way of bringing people into community houses. The resources were seen as empowering both because they were deprofessionalized and owned and run by community people, and also because they were entirely oriented to positive strength-building and skills development (rather than therapy, prevention or risk-factor reduction). The aim was for people to have autonomy and control with regard to both their present and future health and well-being status. Also, they were empowering in that not only were they based on ascertained community need, but also the process of developing them involved continuous consultation and piloting with participants, often over a period of several years, so that many community people had input into the final form they took.

THE SUPERHEALTH LIFESTYLE PROGRAMMES (1974–1989)

Waistline

The first programme to be developed originated in the early days of the BBCP, and was called "Waistline". This programme was initiated in 1974 when a group of 80 or so women who met weekly in the church hall next to the Birkdale Community House, and calling themselves Weightwatchers (even though they were not part of the commercial organization by that name), approached the psychologists associated with the project for assistance in establishing an effective weight-control programme. They said they were having a very enjoyable time socially, but were not losing any weight. At first, this assistance was on a small scale, with a medical student doing a three-month summer project based on R.B. Stuart's early behavioural work on weight control (Stuart, 1967). Then, since the 1975 survey had confirmed weight control as a priority area, it was decided to continue putting an effort into this, and overall about four years were spent in developing and refining the programme. It was then subjected to a quasi-experimental trial, the results of which were published in the American journal *Preventive Medicine* (Raeburn and Atkinson, 1986). All told, about a thousand people went through Waistline during its development and study phases, with the study itself being based on 433 subjects from 68 groups in nine different locations, and involving 23 different group leaders.

The form that Waistline took was of small groups (six to nine people) who met weekly for an hour and a half for 12 weeks. Advertising for the groups was through local community newspapers and community-house publicity systems. Costs were kept as low as possible, with participants paying about a dollar a week to participate. Leaders were "graduates" of previous groups, who were given brief training and then ongoing support and back-up by the psychologists. Usually, leaders were paid a small amount for their work from the participants' contributions, and it was also possible at times to fund the groups through a government-sponsored adult education scheme, so that leaders were able to earn rather more. The aim was to have the course material accessible to all in terms of content, and also to make the financial barriers as small as possible.

The study showed that the programme got results similar to any good behavioural approach—and, at that time, it was generally acknowledged that behavioural approaches were the best for weight control. Overall, an average of 5.6 kg (12.3 lb) was lost by subjects at the end of the 12-week course, and after 12 months, the average amount lost was still 4.3 kg (9.4 lb). However, where Waistline seemed to be different from most other programmes was that not only was it entirely run by lay people in a non-clinical and non-commercial situation, but also it had a very low drop-out rate—only 9–12% on average. This compares with up to 20% for other behavioural weight-control programmes and up to 70% for programmes using other methods (Foreyt and Kondo, 1984; Stunkard and Penick, 1982). Since it can be regarded as a "failure" if a person pulls out of an activity such as weight control, we believe that the community and empowering nature of Waistline was its real strength—people really enjoyed it, found it to be worth while for many reasons, and stuck with it.

This is not the place to go into details of the Waistline programme, but it is worth saying a little about its main features, since the other Superhealth programmes were modelled on it, and because it seemed to work so well.

First, although it was actually started before the 1975 survey results were available, Waistline was clearly in tune with community wishes, as was subsequently ascertained through the needs-assessment surveys.

Second, the long development time, using the process known as "collaborative consultation" (Feldman, 1979), was vital. This involved, in the case of Waistline, the original attempt by the medical student to come up with a programme, consultation with potential participants about this programme, then trying it out, and modifying it accordingly. An "iterative" process of consultation/trying-out/modification went on for several years and, by the time it reached its "final form", Waistline bore little resemblance to its original version. It had truly been developed as a partnership between "the community" and "the experts", combining the best available behavioural weight control technology with the wisdom of community people and participants. This process itself was empowering for participants, since they knew the programme was in a development phase, and that their input would be used for its continuing development.

Third, there were always two agendas in the programme. One was the ostensible one of losing weight. The other was a more hidden one of developing friendship and support, and a sense of strength and self-esteem. Waistline was always seen as a tool for community development. Although weight control as an enterprise has had its critics in recent years, it was always one of the most popular BBCP activities, and was an excellent vehicle to bring people into the project. Many of these people would then stay to participate in other activities, and a number went on to take leadership roles in the project.

Fourth, the emphasis in Waistline was a holistic one, and was concerned with the total development of the person, and all-round positive health, rather than just being exclusively focused on weight. Considerable emphasis was put on exercise, and looking at other dimensions of life. In particular, the social context of the person was given a great deal of attention—that is, how one copes with weight control and health promotion activities in the context of family, social occasions, shopping on a budget, visiting relatives, and so on. Weight issues with children were also covered.

Fifth, most of the session time in Waistline was spent in group discussion, based on brief trigger input material. In general, information about appropriate diet, exercise, potential social blocks, temptation situations, and so on were raised, and then people would spend the time discussing how they would deal with these things in the context of their own lives. In other words, the group process was trusted, and there was a balance between "expert" input, and the wisdom inevitably generated in the group situation. Groups were also active in other ways. For example there would sometimes be role-playing of difficult situations, or actual practice of exercise regimes.

Sixth, "homework" was set each week, based on the material covered in that session. For example, after learning about appropriate aerobic exercise, participants were asked to engage in an exercise they had selected for that week, to give them the opportunity to try it out in their real-life setting. At the start of the next session, each person would report on how they had got on, in both written and verbal form. This, of course, put considerable pressure on people to comply, and ensured that the discussions were well grounded in reality.

Seventh, the generally deprofessionalized nature of the programme, the group leaders who were "peers" of those participating, the ownership of the whole process by the community, and the substantial "content input" by the community both in terms of the development of the course and the actual sessions from week to week, meant that the whole ethos was an empowering one. Also, the emphasis on strength and health-building in a positive way, rather than on "weight" alone, was felt to be empowering.

Unstress

By 1978, it was clear that the Waistline model was working well, and it was decided to set up a second programme on the same general lines. This was eventually called "Unstress", and was an attempt to meet the need found consistently in surveys for something in the stress management area.

Overall, Unstress took about three years of community consultation and pilot testing to develop. It took what was at that time the "best" psychological knowledge about stress management of a cognitive–behavioural variety (since that fitted the theoretical inclinations of the psychologists), and translated this into extremely simple and homely terms, which also seemed to be very powerful. The names and content of the sessions were as follows:

1. Introduction/Pre-Course Evaluation
2. The Mind and Stress (cognition, "awfulizing", life goals)
3. Taking Positive Action (decision-making, immediate goals, persistence)
4. Keep It Simple! (time management, realistic expectations, taking breaks)

5. All in the Family (blaming and resentment, others who block goals, shared family goals)
6. Peace at All Costs? (assertion)
7. Relaxation (muscle-based relaxation)
8. Mental Relaxation (meditation)
9. Nutrition and Fitness (healthy eating, aerobic exercise, sleep)
10. Planning for the Future/Post-Course Evaluation

Unstress took the same general form as Waistline. As can be seen from the list above, it consisted of 10 sessions. These took place once a week for about 90 minutes each. The groups were of five to nine people, led by a lay "graduate" of a previous Unstress course. Materials were available for participants to take away with them from each session, and there was homework and reporting back as for Waistline. Instead of reporting back in terms of weight goals, participants discussed their progress in terms of course goals and life goals. In addition, participants reported back from "lifestyle diaries", kept to record daily relaxation, exercise and other lifestyle habits.

Whereas weight control is, in principle, a conceptually simple area, and easily measurable, stress management is entirely a different matter. In particular, since the aim was to have a deprofessionalized group activity that could be run and attended by virtually anyone, a delicate balance had to be struck between allowing topics to be raised that involved real and difficult life stresses and crises for people, and keeping a level that was positive and readily handled by lay leaders. This was achieved by publicizing Unstress as being concerned with "everyday stress". It was definitely not to be seen as "therapy", nor as a means of dealing with current major life crises. Rather, Unstress was seen as being about generic "skills for living" to deal with present everyday life situations, and with future stresses and strains. For example, one important aspect of Unstress was the learning of what was called "self-relaxation", which included both "physical relaxation" (differential or muscle-based relaxation) and "mental relaxation" (meditation–relaxation, based on Herbert Benson's method; Benson, 1975). As part of their resource kit, participants were given a cassette audiotape with relaxation instructions to practise at home. (Note: this tape has since been independently marketed by one of the research sponsors of the Superhealth programmes, the Mental Health Foundation of New Zealand, and over 20 000 have been distributed throughout New Zealand.) This emphasis on relaxation came from needs assessments, which showed that "tension" was the area most people signing up for Unstress wanted to do something about and, as the results show, there was good success in this area. Another "generic skill" area was based on concepts from Albert Ellis's rational–emotive approach (Ellis and Grieger, 1977). Here, the Ellis concept of "terribilizing" or "catastrophizing" was converted into a New Zealand version of "awfulizing", and it was found that everyone could readily relate to this concept. Also emphasized in the course was the setting of clear personal goals—indeed, the first task in the course was to look at one's overall life goals, and to check whether one was doing what one really wanted to do. Stress, as represented in this course, was seen mainly to do with a lack of clarity about life goals, or having goals that for various reasons were being blocked or otherwise not fulfilled. As can perhaps be seen, the People System model of organizing things around clear goals was here transferred to the personal level!

Blockages to personal goals were often perceived by participants to relate to social factors—family responsibilities, family resistance, lack of opportunities in the community, and so on. Practical solutions to these social aspects were seen as requiring positive action, and assertion and social skills training were areas that were featured in Unstress. Overall lifestyle in terms of eating, exercise, sleep, and other dimensions was also covered, and it was emphasized that one's overall physical and mental condition was important for coping with stress.

These concepts were simple and readily comprehended by anyone. Indeed, the educational level of most of the people attending the programme was modest, with 46% not having obtained the national third year high-school qualification. However, the level of positive satisfaction with the programme was high, and the changes were quite marked (see below).

The measures used to evaluate Unstress covered a range of self-report items, including standardized psychological tests, analogue scales, reports of behavioural activities, satisfaction, tailor-made questions, and so on. Once the programme had achieved its "final form", it was subjected to a quasi-experimental trial, the results of which were published in the *Journal of Community Psychology* (Raeburn et al., 1993). This trial involved 448 subjects in 61 groups in 14 different locations and using 15 different leaders. It spanned a period of five years.

The findings were, in brief, as follows. By the end of the 10-week course, 16% of the participants had dropped out, leaving a study group of 360. On the six psychological tests that were used (e.g. the Spielberger Stait–Trait Anxiety Inventory, and various measures of coping, tension–relaxation and well-being), there were significant positive changes all at the $P<0.0001$ level, with the study group significantly superior to the control group on all counts. For individual goal-setting, the most common goals were to learn to relax, worry less, learn to control events, and be happier, with a range of one to three goals per person. A total of 78% of goals were given ratings of moderate or better progress after the 10 weeks. Measures were also taken of symptoms and behaviours that people hoped the course would improve. The most common of these were tension (94% wanted to change in this area), tension headaches, sleep problems, and drinking too much. All these areas (and others) showed reductions, with "problem gone" or "improved" reported for 85% of those with tension, 73% for tension headaches, 69% for sleep problems and 50% for alcohol use. Another change reported was less tranquillizer use (65% of those who wanted to, cut down). Of smokers, 8% recorded having stopped and 37% said they were smoking less. On more global questions, 96% noticed changes in themselves since starting the course and, of these, 92% said these changes were positive. When asked if their purposes for coming to Unstress had been met, 93% answered affirmatively, The overall satisfaction assessment of the course showed 90% rating it positively.

Follow-up was after 12 months. These data showed that, of the four main "problem" areas, two had improved further since post-course evaluation (sleeping and tension headaches) and, in two, improvements had declined somewhat (tension and drinking). Two-thirds of participants reported that three of the four areas (drinking being the exception) were still better than when they started the course. In response to other questions relating to areas such as current status with regard to mental health, happiness and general ability to handle stress, 96–100% of participants at 12-month follow-up reported that they had changed in positive directions on these dimensions compared with when they started the course. Eighty per cent of participants also gave a positive response for their physical health. In terms of global impression and satisfaction, 83% at 12-month follow-up reported that they were still aware of course-related changes and, of those, 88% perceived the changes as positive. Forty-nine per cent said that they had continued to improve generally since finishing the course, and 86% said the course was still of assistance for their overall coping.

In short, then, the Unstress course seems to have had a significant impact on people's everyday stress levels and coping abilities, and to a great extent these effects were of an enduring nature—for at least a year, anyway. And, obviously, people really liked the course.

Superhealth Basic

By the mid-1980s, it was concluded that the Waistline and Unstress "model" seemed to be one worth pursuing as a more general approach to lifestyle change. It was therefore decided to develop a short (six-week) course of an introductory or "basic" nature, which took the three areas of relaxation, nutrition and aerobic exercise, components common to the two courses so far, and made these the focus of a new "generic" or introductory lifestyle-change course, from which people could then branch out into more "specialist" courses such as Waistline and Unstress. These deliberations led to the formulation of a course called "Superhealth Basic". (Note that in terms of

PCHP and People System philosophy, the "need" for such a course did not arise directly from needs assessments. Rather, it was a "good idea" that occurred as a natural thing to do by the researchers. However, from that point on, there was a great deal of community consultation about the course, which seemed to suggest it was wanted.)

The initial running of Superhealth Basic in community houses met with a positive response. However, it was realized that the necessity to train and support community leaders was becoming a burden with which the small, part-time research team could no longer cope. Thus the idea was floated of replacing trained community leaders with audiotaped input. That is, Super-health would be available as a completely self-contained kit with audiotapes and other materials, and would basically be self-running (even though a "group convener" would be required to turn the audiotapes on and off, and to make the arrangements to ensure that the group ran successfully).

A trial based on 76 people was tentatively done of a taped version of Superhealth Basic (which otherwise had all the structural characteristics of Waistline and Unstress), and it turned out to be both well received and effective (80% said the course had had a positive impact on them and 84% said that the audiotape format should be retained). The evaluations showed that the audiotape version was as effective as a live leader in facilitating behaviour change. So two potential disadvantages of the audiotape format—its "impersonality" and its lack of effectiveness—were not borne out by the evaluations. This theoretically meant that the "sky was the limit" for the community distribution of this programme, and in 1986 funds were obtained from the National Heart Foundation of New Zealand, with support from the Mental Health Foundation of New Zealand, for a research project to develop not only the Superhealth Basic programme as an audiotape-based resource, but also Waistline and Unstress.

To cut a long story short, a quasi-experimental trial was done of the audiotaped version of Superhealth Basic involving 141 people in 19 groups and three conditions (for details, see Raeburn et al., 1994). This showed that there were significant positive behavioural and well-being changes over a wide variety of measures. Also, participants set individual goals (to be more relaxed, to be fitter, to eat healthier food, to lose weight, etc.), and by six weeks, all these had moved 20–43% in a positive direction. Asked to rate the "main effect of the course on you", 91% said "positive" or "very positive". At 12-month follow-up, there were no significant declines on any of the measures showing improvement, and on some measures there were actually gains. Also at follow-up, of the subjects in the main study group, 75% reported improved overall health and 93% positive health behaviour change, both of which were attributed to the course. Ninety per cent said the study had had a positive effect on them, and 100% expressed positive satis-faction with the study.

Eatwell

As mentioned, the principal funder of the latter part of the Superhealth research was the National Heart Foundation of New Zealand. By this time, the role of nutrition in cardiovascular disease was starting to get increased attention. Originally, the intention had been to redevelop Waistline as an audiotape resource as the next phase in the Superhealth research programme. However, at that time (in the mid-1980s) there was controversy around the merits of weight control as an enterprise. For example, there was doubt being raised in the medical literature about the health benefits of weight control, and feminists were questioning whether weight control was a socially desirable activity. These matters put into doubt the wisdom of continuing with Waistline in its original form, and it was therefore decided to consult once again at the community level before proceeding further. As a result of this consultation, plus the current interests of the National Heart Foundation at that time, as well as a growing general community interest in healthy nutrition that had emerged in some of our community surveys, the decision was made to develop a new audiotape programme focused on healthy eating rather than on weight control as such. (We made the assumption that healthy, moderate eating in conjunction with aerobic exercise should tend to "normalize" weight in those who were overweight. However, this assumption was not borne out by the results.)

The name of the new course was "Superhealth Eatwell: A Beginner's Guide to Healthy Eating". It covered six weeks and used a similar taped format to Superhealth Basic. The six session names and their contents were:

1. Introduction (getting to know others in group, outline of course, pre-course evaluation, discussion of healthy diet, goal-setting)
2. Just a Little at a Time (changing food quantities, introducing new foods)
3. Family for Better or Worse (dealing with family resistance or opposition from others to eating habit and food changes)
4. Questions and Answers (experts on the tape answer frequently asked questions; shopping, cooking)
5. Let's Get Physical (exercise, relaxation)
6. Looking Back and Looking Forward (review, how to maintain changes and motivation)

At the heart of the Eatwell course was a "Food Guide" broken down into the main food groups, and consisting of four levels going from the simplest changes to sophisticated changes. Participants located their own "baseline" position on this chart for each food group, and then set goals accordingly, moving gradually from one level to the next in a behavioural "successive approximation" fashion. But equally important as the Food Guide and the setting of individual goals were the support, enthusiasm and fun generated in these groups. Another key aspect was the emphasis on contextual factors such as the family environment. Consideration of a number of issues around culture and food was important, especially given the crucial role of food in different cultures, but this subject is too complex to go into here. Suffice to say that this version of Eatwell was based on a mainstream "European" New Zealand diet, but had the potential to adapt to any kind of diet.

The Eatwell programme, as with the other Superhealth programmes, took some time to develop in a participatory way. Then, once having reached an acceptable "final form", it was subjected to a quasi-experimental trial with 109 participants in 14 groups, including control groups. The results of this are still being written up, but in brief the findings were as follows.

The overall drop-out rate was higher than in previous trials—18%—mainly because two of the groups foundered. (One group was workplace-based, and could not find a time when everyone could meet together, and the other decided that the course was too basic for them.) However, of those groups that remained, the drop-out rate was only 8%. A variety of self-report measures relating to eating behaviour, nutrition, other lifestyle behaviours, and health and well-being were used, as well as physical measures such as weight and blood pressure. (Because we could not find any other studies of community-based healthy eating courses, we were obliged to develop a number of new "eating" measures to suit this situation.) Diaries were also used.

At the end of the six-week course, significant positive changes in a healthy direction ($P<0.0001$) were found in intake of the three food types considered to be most related to health—fats/oils, sugar and salt. There was also a reduction in intake of dairy products and animal protein (thought to be desirable given the New Zealand dairy- and meat-oriented diet), and the consumption of vegetable protein increased. Overall, there was a significant improvement in self-assessed "general eating pattern" in the study group compared with controls. Significant changes in healthy directions were also reported on a number of other measures, including energy levels, exercise and sleep. However, although about half the participants were classified as overweight, there were no significant changes in weight.

At follow-up (nine months), these improvements were maintained at almost the same level as at the six-week evaluation, with some measures slightly (but not significantly) below, and others actually showing further gains. Also, 75–90% of participants reported having made further progress with their Food Guide goals. When asked if they attributed the positive changes in their eating habits to the course, 88% said "Yes". Another interesting finding was that, compared with the six-week post-course evaluation, where the number of significant psychological, health and well-being changes were limited to energy, exercise and sleep, at the nine-month follow-up, there were more such improvements reaching significance, including well-being, mental health and stress, happiness, less tiredness during the day, and overall rated state of health. Unfortunately, there were still no significant changes in weight for those who were overweight. (We feel the added changes that appeared at follow-up are a reflection of the relatively slow psychological and health impact of improvements in eating habits.)

In terms of satisfaction, at the end of the six-week course, 72% answered positively when asked whether they felt Eatwell had met the goals they had when they came to the course, and 83% expressed a positive response when asked about the effect of the course on them. When asked to give their overall impression of Eatwell, 81% said it had been "good", "very good" or "excellent". At nine-month follow-up, these satisfaction measures had actually increased, with 79% attributing an improvement in their eating habits to the course, and 91% reporting an overall positive impression of the course. In addition, 53% said they would be keen to participate in other similar types of Superhealth programmes, and 54% said their overall state of health had improved since doing the course.

Our conclusion from this is that Eatwell was an effective and well-liked programme. As far as we know, it is the first example of a researched, community-based, generic "healthy eating" programme anywhere. What is especially important for a programme such as this, we believe, is not just that it had a positive impact by the end of the course, but that the knowledge and skills learned seemed to go on being of benefit over time, perhaps helping people to change in a permanent fashion. This seems to have been achieved not only by Eatwell, but to some extent by all the Superhealth programmes.

RELATIONSHIP OF THE SUPERHEALTH PROGRAMMES TO PCHP

The programmes described in this chapter may seem more like "conventional" health promotion programmes, and less like "community development", than the other examples we are covering in this book. Also, their emphasis on lifestyle might make them "suspect" in PCHP terms, since the concept of lifestyle has been seen by many in the "new" health promotion as the symbol of old-fashioned, non-empowering and non-holistic health promotion. Do these programmes, then, deserve to be regarded as examples of PCHP? We believe that they do fulfil many of the values and principles of PCHP, and we make this case as follows.

1. People-centredness

The attempt (for the most part, at least) to ground the whole development of the Superhealth programmes in what community people said they wanted, and through the process of participatory consultation to construct these programmes in terms of how the participants see the world, is an example of people-centredness in action.

2. Empowerment

The three dimensions of empowerment of special relevance here are control, strength-building and a resource-based approach. The programmes were based on strongly expressed community wishes, and there was a good deal of community "ownership" and involvement in the developmental process. Once developed, the programmes were available to the communities to use as they wished, typically at no cost or for the cost of materials only. At a more personal level, the programmes were aimed at people developing a sense of personal control over relatively "uncontrollable" life factors (eating habits, external stresses, family and life situations, etc.), and did this in a way that was positive and strength-building. This enabled people to be confident and independent in future situations, an outcome demonstrated by the maintained or improved results at follow-ups 9 or 12 months later.

Another feature of the Superhealth programmes from an empowering perspective was their availability as self-contained resource kits. This seems to us an excellent model for empowerment in health promotion—that is, to have resources available to community people to use as they wish, which they can own, and which are designed to build individual and group strengths.

Finally, to the extent that empowerment and participation are linked, these programmes were very participatory by their nature, and the powerful and positive group processes they engendered were perhaps their most striking feature.

3. Organizational and Community Development

The Superhealth programmes embody elements of community development when they are seen as an integral component of larger community development enterprises, such as the BBCP. For example, they served to bring many people into that project, and also had a strong community network-building function in their own right.

A dimension that is one of the most important features of the Superhealth programmes is that of *group* development. In the Superhealth groups, a powerful sense of friendship was evident, partly because of the intimate nature of the material being covered (so that an ethos of trust and sharing was present), and partly because of the participatory and supportive nature of these groups. Also, the nature of the resource materials was lively, humorous, positive and friendly, so that these elements also lent to the growth of a strong group cohesion.

4. Participation

The Superhealth programmes were designed for people at all levels of society and all backgrounds. They are simple, user-friendly, and capture, we believe, the "true feeling" of people at the community level. And, as is clear from what has already been said, both their development and their process was participatory to a marked degree.

The aim was also achieved of having these activities at such low cost to participants that no one, even the poorest, would be excluded because of unaffordability.

5. Life Quality

The underlying agenda of each programme was with quality of life in all its dimensions. Each programme considered its specific topic area in a wider context of general lifestyle factors, and also of the family and community factors impinging on the person's life. Also relevant to the quality of life dimension was the uncompromisingly positive aspect of the programmes. Even though the trigger for coming to a Superhealth course might have been a "negative" matter such as being overweight or stressed, the approach to dealing with this matter was entirely positive and strength-building.

6. Evaluation

It goes without saying that evaluation was a central component in all that was done here, especially as each programme was developed in a research setting. However, what we hope is apparent is that this evaluation also enhances the health promotion process. It gives the whole enterprise a direction and "edge". It also seems to be rewarding for community participants to be involved in a "research project', especially one that produces such positive results.

In conclusion, then, the Superhealth programmes offer quite a different view of a PCHP approach from the previous example of the community houses, but can still be regarded as being true to PCHP principles. This shows that the same overall organizational structure and values can be used in a variety of ways, to good effect. It is the philosophy, intention and nature of the processes that count, not just the content.

14

CASE STUDIES III
The North Shore Community Health Network* and the Other Way Project

In this chapter, we look at two later examples of the application of the People System approach, and how they fulfil PCHP principles. The first of these, the North Shore Community Health Network, represents perhaps the "loosest" example of the application of a People System/PCHP approach to be given, in that it was set up and run by people who were influenced by a variety of philosophies and approaches, of which the People System was only one. It has been, and remains, a very successful and innovative project, characterized by us as an "Empowering Resource Centre", and has directly or indirectly touched the lives of thousands of people. It is also the only project reported on here that gets a substantial portion of its funding from the public health system, where it comes under the mental health umbrella. The second example, the Other Way Project, at the time of writing is still in a developmental phase. It is also a "free" interpretation of the People System/PCHP approach. The Other Way Project returns to the concept of generic, locality-based community development, but at a more "fundamental" level than the BBCP. Also, two of its primary concerns are with culture and spirituality, matters to which PCHP gives emphasis, but which have not featured prominently in the examples given so far.

---

* We are indebted to Linda Marsh, Carol Ryan, Sue Moore and Barbara Stanley of the North Shore Community Health Network for assisting with the information in the Network section of this chapter.

NORTH SHORE COMMUNITY HEALTH NETWORK
(1983–PRESENT)

In 1983, one of the coordinators of the BBCP, Glennys Adams, left to take a position as coordinator of volunteer services with a community mental health service run by the Auckland Area Health Board, and serving Auckland's North Shore (population about 160 000). With her experience from the BBCP, Glennys soon became dissatisfied with the official model of volunteer help in use at that time, and determined to take a more "community development" and "self-reliance" approach. To do this, she gradually moved towards establishing a centre where strength-building courses and programmes, together with support from peers, were available. This in turn meant that such "resources" existed not only for those who had recently left the treatment service, but also for anybody who felt they could benefit by participation in activities of a "psycho-educational" or support nature. Thus, the resource centre started to evolve towards being a "primary prevention" or "mental health promotion" centre and its "general" or non-client dimension grew to be its primary emphasis. A listing of the aims of the volunteers presented at a public meeting in 1983 gives a flavour of this new emphasis.

- To promote positive mental health within the community.
- To work alongside the community to identify mental health needs.
- To be a link between community groups and professionals and to act as advocates to ensure that "grass-roots" community mental health needs are given a voice.
- To ensure that "mental health" is represented and acknowledged as an integral part of all community health endeavours (holistic approach).

In 1984, another coordinator was appointed, and the organization declared its existence as an independent, recognizable entity by forming itself into an incorporated society, called the North Shore Community Health Network, Inc. (hereafter called the "Network"). This is a remarkable organization because, although the staff are mainly paid by the public health service, the control of the organization, through the elected committee, is in the hands of community people, some professional, some not. This unlikely "balance" of official/non-official power structures has existed successfully since that time, largely because of the shared vision and positive "culture" of the whole endeavour. And, although there have been periods when official funding has been under threat, the organizational structure itself has continued to work well. After two moves, the resource centre was finally located (in 1986) on the grounds of North Shore Hospital in a free-standing, ordinary brick house facing on to a main thoroughfare street, and made available to the Network by the hospital for a peppercorn rental. This location was a symbol of the organizational structure of the project. It was, on the one hand, still part of the public health system, with the majority of its funding coming from the mental health services. On the other hand, it had a substantial measure of independence, with many of its activities not directly under the control of the health system, and some of its funding coming from sources other than the mental health service.

Since the centre was established, the whole New Zealand health system has been through radical changes in its funding and organizational structure, and the funding of the centre is now mainly on a contestable contract basis, which in many respects suits the autonomy of the centre better. However, since it also has to be seen to be providing needed "services" in a tight financial climate, some of its flexibility to do "health promotion" has been limited. But, to the extent that some of its funds come from sources other than the public health sector, it has room for setting its own agendas.

As we say, we (the authors) call this enterprise an "Empowering Resource Centre" (ERC). Although this is not a term used by the organization itself, we feel it sums up the centre's role from a PCHP perspective. That is, it functions primarily as a multidimensional resource and support centre to community groups (ranging from individuals and families, through self-help groups, to whole communities) wanting to take self-determined action in a wide variety of health, mental health, personal development and community development areas. At the time of writing, the Network has six paid part-time staff members (3.7 full-time equivalents) whose roles are labelled as community project coordinator, self-help group coordinator/community liaison, resource coordinator/community liaison, financial administrator/secretary and reception/support worker. There are also 14 casual staff and 20 voluntary workers. The bulk of the activities relate to the "self-help" area, especially to self-help and support groups. However, there are many other activities and functions, covering information, knowledge, skills, consultancy, organizational development, community development, premises, facilities such as computers and photocopying, advocacy and various other "resources". The Network operates broadly within a PCHP philosophy, with an emphasis on empowerment and an "Ottawa Charter" perspective. This may be seen from its current constitutional statement of objectives, which reads:

(a) To develop and utilize resources in the communities on the North Shore to meet the mental health needs of these communities (hereinafter called "the communities") and to actively work towards the prevention of mental illness.

(b) To provide a framework for the co-ordination of activities and facilities designed to promote the well-being of the communities.
(c) To ensure the activities and facilities are related to the health needs of the communities.
(d) To provide support, guidance and education for members who endeavour to achieve the objectives of this society.
(e) To promote educational opportunities for individuals, families and groups to develop their own learning and well-being and to find their own solutions with self-reliance and neighbourly help.
(f) To identify and liaise with appropriate community groups, statutory and professional agencies based in the communities.
(g) To facilitate ongoing evaluation of all the society's activities.
(h) To be open to affiliation with any other society, body or organizations having objectives similar or ancillary to the objects of this society within these Rules.

The mission statement of the centre is to "enable people to have greater choice in determining their own wellbeing and health by providing information, resources and networks of support", and their current stated philosophy is as follows:

We, the Network acknowledge the relevance of the Treaty of Waitangi (*Tiriti O Waitangi*) and the Maori people as *Tangata Whenua* in Aotearoa.
   The focus of the Network is to enable people to achieve health.
   We see health as a state of physical, social, emotional, cultural and spiritual well-being which is influenced by social, cultural, economic, personal and political factors.
   For health to be achieved, all these factors need to be addressed.
   Therefore the Network's involvement in health promotion is to empower communities to have more influence on the factors that determine their health.
   We believe that when communities are empowered, people are more able to control their own endeavours and destinies.

As the use of goals might suggest, the Network's *modus operandi* is based broadly on the People System approach to organization. However, it is an example of a very flexible application of this system. While the managers of the organization took the People System type of approach as their broad starting point, they interpreted it to suit their own values and way of looking at things. For example, needs assessment has always been an area of difficulty for this organization. Because it serves such a large population, the centre is more of a regional resource facility than a local, community-scale enterprise. It is therefore difficult to "do a survey" to determine the overall needs of this population. At the same time, the Network has a strong commitment to the principle of needs assessment, and has a number of less formal ways of ascertaining needs.

Since the Network is included here as an example of a PCHP project, there may be some question as to whether it legitimately belongs in this framework. What follows is a brief analysis of how it does relate to PCHP principles.

1. People-centredness

The Network is strongly committed to a "people perspective", rather than to a professional one, and that consideration probably exceeds all others. Its aim is to honour the values and wishes of ordinary people, especially those "in need", and to work by their agendas. Its orientation is a community one, not an institutional one, and there are strong linkages with community people and groups throughout the whole district.

As may be seen from the mission statement, there is also a strong commitment to a cultural perspective, in particular a bicultural one, which recognizes the equal roles and rights of the two main population groups in New Zealand, Maori and *Pakeha*.

In terms of professional roles, certainly the type of role assumed by the paid staff based in the centre is a facilitatory one. They are very aware of the principles of empowerment and facilitation, and spend a good deal of time discussing their roles, attending workshops on the topic, and so on. They certainly acknowledge that the "jpf's" ("just plain folks") are in charge, and that their role as staff is simply to facilitate, resource, support and sometimes advocate on behalf of the aspirations and activities of those people.

2. Empowerment

The Network has always had empowerment as its number one philosophical principle. Empowerment is seen primarily in terms of self-empowerment, that is, the psychological power and potential for self-development that is available through supportive groups. But empowerment for the Network has also had a "political" aspect to it as well. Here is how one of the staff members represented the Network's approach to empowerment, after she attended a 1993 conference in Australia on the topic of "Social change, community empowerment, and enablement". In this passage, she uses the term "groking", borrowed from science fiction writer Isaac Asimov:

> "Groking" as I use it, is a group process which involves people who share a common problem or concern and are closely culturally matched.
> [One example] could be a group of [Australian] aboriginal women concerned about the sexual abuse of their children within a geographical community. Another [example] could be a group of leaders concerned about aboriginal deaths in custody. Group members would require a passionate concern or intense anger and a determination to do something. The process inevitably involves strong emotions and a subjective approach.

(The very antithesis of the rationality of a psychological approach.) Conflict is probable as members of the group seek to understand and clarify the nature of the problem and identify possible actions/strategies for change. If they discover factors that identify a structural or political base to the problem rather than ascribing difficulties to personal inadequacy, members feel empowered. This process of talking/groking together is likely to take a long time . . .

The Community Support projects at North Shore Network are . . . examples of this approach. (Adams, 1993, p. 4)

As can be seen, empowerment is represented here as a matter of having control over the process of doing something about a perceived problem that has a strong emotional or distress component, and realizing that it is a structural rather than personal matter. After having conceptualized the problem and then feeling strong enough to do something about it, the group takes its own action, with or without the assistance of a "professional ally". This is where the availability of an accessible range of knowledge and other resources is especially helpful. Through this process comes a sense of growing strength and empowerment, as skills are developed to take the appropriate action, and social bonds are cemented.

From an overall organizational perspective, there is also an empowerment or control dimension too, since the Network is run by a committee, and anyone can potentially be elected on to this committee, and help set policy. Similarly, while in the past there were mental health professionals on the staff, currently none has that background, which shows the capacity of "community people" to become leaders through a process of empowerment, as described by Kieffer (1984)—see Chapter 5.

3. Organizational and Community Development

The Network puts a high value on its organizational aspect, and uses an annual goal structure around which to focus its activities. It is clear that one of the reasons the Network has been able to survive in spite of a precarious health system environment is that it has been so well organized and managed. In particular, its record and documentation systems are outstanding, and these have been used repeatedly to demonstrate to officialdom and others that the Network makes a major contribution, and that it is extremely well run and accountable.

As far as community development is concerned, this area occupies about a third of staff time and project resources. The Network has been involved in a number of projects on a consultancy basis, notably with several community houses, and with a major Maori project. It has also assisted with a number of surveys, and has had a role with the Other Way Project, discussed in the final part of this chapter.

4. Participation

The Network is clearly a participatory project, in the sense that its intention is to involve anyone and everyone who feels that personal and community development are relevant to them, and that community people are involved in all aspects of the organization. As far as possible, the agendas are set by community people rather than by professionals, and the activities are generally of a "popular" and accessible nature oriented to attracting a wide sector of the population. Inevitably, as in all such projects, the majority of participants are female, and in spite of efforts to promote men's activities, only about 6% of participants in overall Network activities are male. The effort to make biculturalism a principal emphasis also means that Maori are encouraged to participate, although this in practice tends to mean support and resources for their own self-determined, within-culture groupings, rather than a more general participation.

5. Life Quality

In so far as quality of life is a subjectively experienced thing—which is the stance we have taken—then clearly the spectrum of activities that come under the concept of "mental health" as dealt with by the Network are relevant to quality of life. Taken overall, it may be seen that the transcendent goal of the Network is the enhancement of quality of life—that is, of positively experienced well-being and of the ability to participate in life's opportunities by as many people in its district as possible.

This view is reinforced by the Network's adoption of the Ottawa Charter as a primary guiding document, which means that a broad ecological viewpoint is taken, including political, environmental, community, social and personal dimensions. Its commitment to positivity also reflects this, and to the visitor, this positivity—the fun, the laughter, the goodwill and kindness—which permeates the whole atmosphere of the operation, is perhaps its most striking aspect, and is a living illustration of what quality of life means.

One must add to this another dimension, which has not come up to any extent in relation to the other projects we have discussed, and that is the transpersonal or spiritual dimension. Increasingly, this is an explicit aspect of the Network's activities, in response to what is perceived by the staff as a strong interest in the community.

6. Evaluation

Evaluation and accountability are highly valued in the Network. The main mechanism by which these are accomplished is by an exact record of outputs in various areas, including numbers participating in groups and activities. A modified form of the Impact Questionnaire (Chapter 11) is also used in each group. For example, in 1996, 54 groups were supported by the Network. One of these is "New Outlook", a support group for older women. The 1996 evaluative summary for this group reads:

> Many of the women [entering the group] reported feeling isolated or depressed. Some were on medication for depression. The group meets with two Facilitators for two hours a week and continued to meet over the holidays by themselves. There are 20 women in the group. [Using the Impact Questionnaire, the following was found:]
>
> 100% stated that the group had helped them cope or manage better
> 94% reported increased wellbeing and happiness during the group
> 67% reported improvement in physical health which they attributed to the group
> 48% stated that they would have used counselling services but for the group
> 26% stated they would have used prescribed drugs but for the group
> 15% stated they would have used hospital services but for the group

In conclusion, then, it can be said that the North Shore Community Health Network is an illustration of what is possible with a PCHP approach within the constraints of a public health service, and with a "free interpretation" of both the philosophy and practice. Its "empowering resource" approach is one that can be used in virtually any setting for any purpose, and provides, we believe, a good model for other such enterprises. It uses a number of elements of the People System of organization, but has made its own adaptation of that approach. The healthiness and impact of what has been achieved is clear from the support it receives from both the community and the public health sector, and from the evaluations that have been done.

THE OTHER WAY PROJECT (1993–PRESENT)

For our final case study, we wish to include a project that is, at the time of writing, still in a developmental phase. This enables us to show how a PCHP/People System approach is being used right now, and how one can use this approach to guide the formation of a project. Indeed, since the example given here is attempting to be true to the principles of allowing the community to determine the direction of things, it is by no means clear what the final form of this project will be. In its short life, it has already made some fundamental changes in emphasis and strategy to reflect both changing societal realities (notably a rapid change in New Zealand's unemployment situation), and an emerging sense from the community that the original strategies intended for the project were not going to work, and needed redirecting. At the same time, there is also the feeling that this project is moving right to the heart of what its community wants.

In the New Zealand of the early 1990s, the single greatest social problem was recognized as being unemployment, the result of decades of recession, then, since 1984, of economic restructuring by successive governments along monetarist lines. Unemployment had grown for more than a decade from previously low levels to about 12% of the workforce. It has now, however, declined to about 6%, although a fluctuating course is anticipated.

The social and health costs of unemployment are widely acknowledged (e.g. Bethwaite et al., 1990). In the New Zealand of the 1980s and early 1990s, these effects seemed especially acute, perhaps because substantial unemployment had hitherto been a relatively unknown phenomenon. Unfortunately, even though the official employment statistics now look better, many of these effects linger on. Much of the work that has been created is low paid, and also, the social welfare benefits of those not in the workforce have been significantly reduced, creating a permanent underclass. In a decade or so, New Zealand went from one of the most equitable societies in the developed world, with little overt poverty, to a society with one of the largest disparities between rich and poor. Paralleling this reality is the fact that rates of homicide, violent crime, rape and other such offences have gone from some of the lowest in the world to some of the highest. At present, New Zealand has the highest recorded rate of youth suicide in the Western world.

These traumatic effects of unemployment and radical economic restructuring in a once cosy welfare state (New Zealand introduced the world's first welfare state system in the 1930s, and in the 1950s was ranked the third richest country in the world after the US and Canada) were not acknowledged by the governments of either the left or right during a period now characterized as a "revolution" in New Zealand. Indeed, the restructuring seemed to be done in an especially heartless and aggressive manner, the philosophy of its architects apparently being to stun the population with such major and rapid change that they did not have time to take stock and protest. This impression of government ruthlessness was strengthened by successive cuts in welfare benefits, putting even further stress on an impoverished and demoralized sector of the population. For the first time in New Zealand, genuine poverty was evident, with children going without food, and the emergence of "food banks" in most centres. In general, there appeared to be a political climate of indifference or even antagonism toward the poor and unemployed, with little being done to plan for unemployment at the community level, apart from some government work schemes. Such planning still seems necessary, given the observation that modern economies seem to produce a permanent and substantial sector of the adult population who are not in full or even part-time paid employment.

It was against a background of concern with the health, mental health and social consequences of unemployment in the New Zealand of the early 1990s that the concept of the Other Way Project arose. Literally, the name means "there has to be another way" than the one that was evident at that time, which seemed to be producing so many disempowered, unhappy and health-threatened people in the community, with virtually nothing official being done about it. And, in spite of the fact that unemployment has dropped significantly for the time being, there is no guarantee that this is permanent, and there is a strong residual distrust of government in terms of their capacity to "care".

What the idea for the Other Way Project also highlighted was the fact that, in any given community, there are not only those who are "unemployed", as that term is usually understood, but also many others who are around during the day, and typically not in full-time work. Apart from school-aged children, such people include non-working parents, the retired and elderly, those on benefits, the ill and disabled, and a variety of others. These people were also of interest here. As unemployment became less of an issue in New Zealand, the needs of these other groups came increasingly into focus. There was no ready label for this heterogeneous group, so we have given them the name of "People Around in Communities Every Day", or "PACED".

However, the first ideas for, and research on, the Other Way Project took place during the period of peak unemployment. The overall concept of the Other Way Project as it was understood at that time is given below in the form of excerpts from a discussion document put out in 1992. As can be seen, this outline is almost a summary of what this book is about.

This project represents a first small effort to develop a model for "another way" for [those in a given locality-based community who are unemployed and those adults not otherwise in the formal, full-time workforce]. The aim is to develop a coordinated, participatory, community-controlled system in communities dedicated to the wellbeing and life satisfaction of this substantial population . . .

The key to this project is its organizational framework at the community level. It is intended to base this on a participatory community development system used in New Zealand over the past 20 years, and which has proved itself in a series of research projects to be effective in enabling communities to work on their own needs and wellbeing. Called the People System, it . . . is based on needs/wishes assessment, community control and evaluation. In this project, it is intended that the following steps be followed:

(1) In each community, a community-based resource centre is established, akin to a community house. Initially, this would be staffed by project workers funded by research grants and other such monies. Later, the centre would be staffed by local people and be self-supporting. What follows is then organized through this centre.

(2) The population of interest is defined (e.g. anyone who has finished school and is not in full-time employment), and then is systematically surveyed to find out what they would like for themselves while not in the workforce. (The domain of the survey would be carefully outlined so that aspirations were within a realistic and attainable framework.)

(3) The needs/wishes of the population of interest are then studied in consultation with that population, so that priorities are determined, and overall and realistic project goals can be set. These goals would have a variety of aims:
  (i) They would be aimed at the development of constructive activities which people would find a satisfying and fulfilling way of using their time, and which may or may not generate income . . .
  (ii) They would permit an orderly development in terms of priorities and resource availability, and each major activity area would be organized as its own semi-autonomous sub-project, with its own goals and management.
  (iii) The goals provide the framework for the evaluation procedures, both for process (management-oriented) reviews and outcome evaluations to determine whether community needs/wishes are being met, and to ascertain the overall impact of the project on community wellbeing.
(4) A local community-controlled organizational structure would be set up for the project, along the lines of the most successful and democratic community houses.
(5) Resource planning for the project would be undertaken, with the aims of making each project self-sufficient.
(6) All activities would be kept under constant review by the project coordinators and the community at large . . . so that all activities proceed in an optimal fashion, and so that there is a forum for tackling generic issues of concern to the project and the community. Overall, the aim would be to have a very well run organization with high morale, high participation rates and high participant satisfaction.
(7) At the end of each year, a formal goal-review and goal-setting exercise would be held, to determine overall progress and status over the year just past, and to establish priorities and goals for the next year. This would be done in a consultative manner involving the community, and there would also be public reports about the project's activities and outcomes associated with this "outcome evaluation" exercise.

. . . The aims of the way of working here are threefold. One is that we believe that the most important route to life satisfaction is when people feel they are engaged in worthwhile activities in which they have a great deal of interest, which they value, and which they feel contribute to themselves and their community. Normally, paid work provides much of these things—here, we are attempting to provide similar satisfactions outside the traditional paid work situation. Second, the "hidden agenda" behind all activities is that of building a sense of support and community. That is, not only do worthwhile activities have a value in their own right, but they also help to develop bonds between people when they are working on common goals together. This community/social development aspect is at the heart of this project. Third, the whole basis of the way of working here is toward people feeling they have a measure of control and mastery over their lives. Not only will they be able to take part in activities of their own choosing, and for which they can gain a sense of mastery and accomplishment, but the collective nature of the enterprise will give a sense of "the community" being in charge of its own destiny. In addition—and this is the key to the People System approach—the whole structure is under the control of the local community and guided by its needs and wishes. Such collective, community-controlled working also means that the community is able to speak with a common voice, which makes it a powerful entity on the political front. If people speak with one voice, then politicians have to listen. (Raeburn, 1992)

Clearly, the Other Way Project attempts to encapsulate much of what we have been talking about in this book. However, the alert reader will perhaps have picked up a basic flaw in what is being proposed here—that is, the whole enterprise has been dreamed up by outsiders, and felt to be a "good" idea for communities, rather than coming out of expressed community "need".

This issue—of introducing an intervention or idea into a community that has not asked for it—is a constant conundrum in community work. More often than not, such "good ideas" will come from someone who sees a community issue, and perhaps a way of dealing with it, but which has not been seen or asked for by that community. At the same time, a good idea is a good idea, especially if the intention is the overall benefit of the community, and the aims of community control and self-determination remain uppermost.

So the way we see to resolving this is by taking a very gradual approach, which begins with informal discussions in the community with key people, and then continues to check out in a very unobtrusive way the feeling of ordinary community people about what is proposed. And, throughout this process, one must be committed either to withdrawing, or completely changing the idea, as reactions and suggestions are made.

The initial plan was to try out the Other Way Project in two communities, Thames and Northcote. The reason for doing this was that two Masters students taking a course in community development and health promotion with John Raeburn in 1994 became interested in the Other Way Project for their own communities, and decided to do their theses in this area. Thames is a provincial service town of about 6000 people 100 km south-east of Auckland, with a relatively high level of industry. Northcote is an old established suburb of about 12 000 people just north of Auckland's harbour bridge. Each student decided to engage in an initial checking-out and needs-assessment process in their communities, using different methodologies and slightly different populations. In Thames, the population of interest was the "unemployed", whereas in Northcote, the population was of any post-school teenagers or adults not in the full-time workforce (i.e. the "PACED" population, including people working less than half-time).

So, was the Other Way Project something that these communities felt they wanted?

In Thames, several focus groups were set up involving health and social service workers, youth workers, agencies such as green dollar (bartering) cooperatives, county councillors and unemployed people. These groups provided a setting for initial discussions about the concept, and to construct an appropriate survey form. The response to the concept among these people was generally positive. These forums were followed by a random survey using rapid ethnographic assessment methodology with 140 unemployed people aged between 16 and 60. Of these, 100% said they thought the project sounded like a good idea, with 90% saying they would like to be part of the project in some shape or form. Most (94%) felt that eventually the project should be open to people of all ages and backgrounds. A clear set of activity preferences emerged, with the top ones being learning a skill or hobby (30%), first aid training and caring for the sick (27%), learning about the law and one's legal rights (22%), learning how to grow one's own food (20%), and increasing self-confidence and self-esteem (16%) (Battisti, 1995).

In Northcote, there was initially a series of in-depth, semi-structured interviews with 20 key people such as school principals, Maori leaders, the police, social service agency workers, youth workers, and so on. A majority (13) of these 20 people expressed support for the project. Two random surveys then followed, a general one of 230 households meeting the PACED criterion throughout the whole of Northcote, and a more focused survey of 56 households in Onepoto, which is a socially distinct enclave of about 1200 people within Northcote. Onepoto is especially notable for its cultural mix, with approximately 30% being Maori, 50% of Pacific Island origin, and 20% European. It also has a higher unemployment rate than the more white, middle-class surrounding area of Northcote.

Both Northcote surveys showed a high level of support for the concept of the Other Way Project. In the larger survey, 80% expressed support for the concept, and the same percentage expressed an interest in participation. Priority areas in terms of personal expressions of interest were job training (90% expressing an interest for themselves), personal development (85%), parent education (79%), more recreational facilities (76%), more opportunity to get together with other local residents (75%), and opportunities to contribute to the community (75%).

In the Onepoto survey, there was even higher support for the project, with 82% expressing support for the concept, and an astonishing 93% saying they would like to be involved in some way. (Previous experience with such surveys shows that such expressed intentions are a reasonable indicator of what will actually take place, provided the project is well implemented.) The pattern of preferences was somewhat different in the Onepoto survey, with educational and skill classes being the top priority (98% expressing personal interest), followed by job training facilities (82%), opportunities to contribute to the community (70%), parent education (67% of parents), and opportunities to get together with other people (64%) (Khoshkhoo, 1996).

In addition to the "activity" and "facility" interests shown in these survey results, there are two important items relevant to a community-building dimension. One is the expressed wish of people to contribute to the community, and the other is the wish to have opportunities to get together with others in the community. As is noted in Chapter 15, many of us simply do not know what other people are thinking and feeling. In spite of the supposed alienation and non-community nature of modern society, there still appears to be for many people a desire to be involved in their local community in a significant way.

We do not have space here to do justice to what has happened since these surveys. In so far as Thames is concerned, the student who did the research, and who was going to continue to spearhead the project there, had to return to the US for domestic reasons, so that project has not gone any further. In Northcote, however, there has been continuing development. We will talk about this briefly now.

In 1996, a research grant was obtained from the Health Research Council of New Zealand to take the Other Way Project in Northcote to its next stage. The grant proposal was difficult to write, since it could not specify exactly what would happen in the project beyond its involving a broad community development process within a People System framework. However, it did state that the intention was to test out the setting up of a street-based programme, called the Street Activation Project. This project would seek "activators" in each of the streets of Onepoto to organize discussions in their streets of the survey findings, from which suggestions would hopefully be made about how to proceed. The aims of this were not just to get useful information, but equally to foster bonds between people at the local street level, and to generate a sense of ownership of the project and energy for action. From a research perspective, the aim was to develop and evaluate an organizational system that would support and facilitate such street-based development, and then extend this to the whole of Northcote. Part of the research was also to do with the development of "community-friendly" evaluative indicators for this type of project, to determine its impact on the quality of life, health and well-being of the community in an unobtrusive and meaningful way, and in a way that was controlled and deemed to be useful by the community.

The grant permitted the two-year funding of a coordinator position, which was filled by Jane West, a local resident in Onepoto, Chair of the local school board, systems consultant, and well-respected person in the community. Jane is a Maori of Ngati Whatua descent, which gives her a local tribal identity. The base for the project is at the Onepoto Awhina, the Northcote Community House, which adjoins the Onepoto area. The Awhina is strategically located in the grounds of the Northcote Shopping Centre, which also has a role in the Northcote Other Way Project (see listing of activities below). In the near future, an incorporated society is to be set up as a framework for the Other Way Project in Northcote.

So, how has the project gone to date? On one level, very well. It is clear that the community was initially suspicious of what was going on, especially as they had been over-researched, and had had bad experiences as a result of that. But, as trust has built with the coordinator, and it is realized that they, the community, are to be in control of what is going on, then there has been a growing momentum of support and involvement. However, as perhaps we should have predicted, the "plan" outlined in the research grant for the Street Activation Project was amiss, in spite of the fact it evolved from almost two years of discussion in the community. Although there was some support for the street activation approach, after various attempts to get it going, it was clear it was not going to work. Mainly, the reason for this seemed to be that it was "too soon"—that the level of trust and stability required for people to have such close relationships with their neighbours was not yet there. As a result, there has been a return to the more conventional "subproject" approach we described previously for the BBCP—that is, where groups of people, not necessarily in the same street, but in reasonable neighbourhood proximity, get together around needs-based goals to participate in activities of common interest to them. However, the approach to this in Northcote has been adapted to fit the "culture" of the area, the result of discussion and listening at street level. The term that Jane West uses for these subprojects is "vehicles"—an approximate English rendering of the Maori word *waka* or canoe—a coordinated entity going somewhere, with a lot of people on board.

These vehicles have their origins in the needs-assessment information from the surveys, and do what we mentioned previously as being one of the "arts" of this kind of community development work. That is, they translate the formal needs-assessment information into activities and projects that are exactly attuned to what the local people in that community want, and which they will take part in and "own". This process began with a formal presentation of the actual thesis containing the survey results to the community at a ceremony at the Onepoto Awhina, opened by a Maori elder from the local *marae* (meeting house and sacred ground). Since then, the thesis has been well read and discussed in the community. (That copy of the thesis is now covered in tea and coffee stains!) Given the gap between the survey period and the discussion of the results in the community (almost three years), some of the information was out of date, especially that relating to the acute unemployment situation. There was also some feeling in the community that the researchers had been too slow in getting back to the community with the results. It was quite clear that people had not forgotten the research. Even though they had supported it initially, they were starting to put it in the same category as the rest of what they regarded as exploitative research— where experts come in to do surveys, promise the world, and then are never seen again.

We mention these matters because it is vital to be aware of them in this sort of environment. It is easy for researchers to see the community as an anonymous entity on which research has no discernible impact. The contrary is true. In fact, "research" can be seen as an intervention in a community—the community is changed by it. Some research can cause ripples for years afterwards, especially in a community like Onepoto, where memories are long, and a climate of cynicism about such things can easily develop—with much justification!

Notwithstanding this slow start, it is clear that the low-key approach adopted by Jane West, the esteem in which she is held in the community, and her understanding of systems processes are combining to make the project a promising one.

There are, at the time of writing, five "vehicles" in active operation. These consist of projects to do with (1) backyard cooperative gardens, (2) the Northcote Shopping Centre and its future development, (3) a community tools scheme, (4) ethnic arts and crafts workers, and (5) *whanau* (extended family) support. The organization is about to be incorporated, and an evaluative indicators research study has begun. Considerable effort was made to set up the Street Activation Project, but this has now been discontinued. Regular review meetings have begun, and a group of residents has formed as a core group to steer the overall project.

To end this account, and to bring it up to the moment of sending this book off to the publisher, we have asked Jane West if she would describe here her perception of the project. In particular, we have asked her to say something about how she sees where the project is at the moment (especially with regard to the "vehicles"), how she views the People System type of approach, how she sees the issues of culture and spirituality in relation to this project, and her predictions for the future. Here is what Jane has written. (Note: The introductory passages in Maori are Jane's placing of herself in terms of location and tribal affiliation, and her greetings to you, the reader. She prefers that these not be translated.)

> *Ko Jane West te ingoa,*
> *Ko Tauwhare te Maunga*
> *Ko Kaipara te Moana, Ko Waipatukohu te Awa*
> *Ko Whiti te Ra te Whare, Ko Reweti te Marae*
> *Ko Te Taou te Hapu*
> *Ko Ngati-Whatua te Iwi*

Kia ora. Ka nui te mihimihi kia koutou. No reira, tena koutou, tena koutou, tena koutou katoa. I take this opportunity to introduce myself to readers before I share with you the basis of my *whakaaro* (purpose) in having a part in the Other Way Project.

New Zealand has slowly been losing something fundamental which a number of sectors of our society now recognize as being at risk, namely a sense of family and of belonging together. We all have an expectation that we can contribute to our own well-being and that of our families, and in cases of genuine need, such well-being would be met collectively by the community at large. The introduction of the welfare system had its purpose from this fundamental credo, as has the movement of community development, which could well be construed as the attempt to "return to the old". In this approach, people are living entities, open to change and a free interpretation of how they view themselves and others, their concerns and/or initiative, in whatever they view as their "community". *A founding Golden Rule—this should never be interpreted for them.*

For my part, this golden rule has been the *kaupapa* (fleets [as of canoes], platform) of the Other Way Project. To achieve clarity in adhering to the *kaupapa* is what, in fact, determined the People System of organization for this project. More importantly, it dictated what was to be attempted, its timing, the order of things, and to what level of satisfaction and/or conclusion. The project's organization, its scope and its delivery mode were also easily identified from the needs-assessment information. It ensured that any action had its origins deriving directly from the community, yet it was flexible enough to be inclusive, giving choices of participation levels, in terms of both interest and extent of participation. Once the project started, while being mindful of not trying to dictate how information was gathered, an "open door" policy to ideas and activities was adopted. This created some issues for the ongoing consultation processes, in reference to location, timing and substance. However such problems were minimized with the introduction of the "vehicles" approach as a means of individually focusing on issues of interest while also being in a collective environment.

The "vehicles" approach, realized from the project's wider *kaupapa*—as a fleet of *waka* (canoes) acting in a "platform" sense—provides choice, while also identifying indicators to determine the project's potential for future application. Each "vehicle" has physical "time and labour" elements [e.g. setting up and growing cooperative backyard gardens], encouraging people to follow through on their decision/desire to participate in a hands-on manner. This was a paramount consideration and its wisdom is now being evidenced in that participants now have a real vision of their potential, both positive and negative. More importantly, practical outcomes demonstrating change can be readily witnessed. Though the project has a research element, the needs assessment which gave birth to the project's concept has, in itself, created change. What is positive about the Other Way Project's intervention *per se* is that the "living elements" [that is, significant parts of people's lives] entrusted as a "gift" to the needs assessment and the project team are being honoured, and are being responded to in a fashion which is conducive to the nature of the community.

The above effectively sets the environment for positive empowerment through participation. I stress these words, as the natural consequence of participating in something which primarily comes from the heart's wish list is empowerment in the truest sense. I consider much of the project, including its indicators and measurements, to be based on elements of common sense. It is the external factors of academic and analytical skills that make, in my opinion, community development debatedly the contribution of the century. Without such an approach, there is a tendency to miss the basics of the living elements which give us our holistic well-being. We either take them for granted or misinterpret them. To take others for granted, and/or misinterpret their feelings and concerns, puts you into a category which is not conducive to people-orientated empowerment.

The Other Way Project continues to work through raising issues with the community being at the forefront, as any changes and initiatives must not only include the very people they affect, but also be designed and driven by those people, *as of right*.

Discussions with the people at street level in the community identified that the reasons for desired participation were both in the singular and in the plural. That is, the reasons were "for growth" of both the individual and/or the family. Throughout the project's first year, it became apparent that participation was based on the beforementioned "living elements" which are collective to all of us, however we may express them differently. For myself, the same applies when I refer to community development. What naturally comes to mind is "developing holistic well-being for growth". To achieve holistic well-being is the ultimate, and in attempting its achievement with others, my *Tikanga Maori* [Maori culture] enhances me and directs me therein. The *tapu* (sacred) elements of my *whaakaro* (purpose) direct my responses accordingly in my conduct and attitude, and in the relationships that are created through anything that is undertaken. It can be equated to my code of conduct, which gives me strength and discipline in the sense of respecting others. *Tapu* principles are far-reaching, and are more than the restrictive *tapu* that most are familiar with. It also relates to value, dignity and worth "by reason of being". It involves our relationships with others and with other created things. For the project, it is seen through the links between people (as in personal), with land/location and with the wider people. To achieve clarity in such elements is to achieve the order of things in life.

In conclusion, and in relation to the project, I have no predictions other than to say the project is aptly named. By founding the project on things that are intrinsic to us, and being inclusive as of right, while according dignity that naturally commands respect towards the people participating in the things attempted therein, it is indeed the "other way"!

15

TOWARDS A PCHP SOCIETY

In this final chapter, we want to indulge ourselves by providing our vision of what an ideal society might be like based on PCHP principles.

This vision involves a society built on the principles of "true democracy" and "government from the periphery". Our brief foray into fantasy here does not claim to have worked through all the political and economic details, and no doubt there will be many who, from their ivory or glass towers, will say this would not work. But given the fact that most economists and politicians cannot agree on even the most basic fundamentals, it seems to us there is at least some scope for a "vision" such as the one we present here. And, if there is a will, ways will always be found. We are realistic enough, however, to concede that there is not likely to be much official will for this, much less the way!

To present this, we would like to return to our original breakdown of the mnemonic "PEOPLE", and extend the concepts from the domain of health promotion and local community to society at large. But, before we do this, some preliminary words.

To us, perhaps the most inspirational thing we encountered while writing this book was the information about grass-roots movements in developing countries. As the title of Durning's (1989) Worldwatch article says, these movements may be "our best hope for global prosperity and ecology", and perhaps one could add "and quality of life". What these movements show is that, in spite of often powerful opposition from governments and exploitative corporate and other interests, people can nevertheless determine their own destinies, and improve their own quality of life in dramatic ways. And undoubtedly the key to this is what, for want of a better term, we have called "empowerment". That is, people articulate what they want for themselves, then set about in a collective and community-based way to develop their own and their community's strengths and resources. By this means, the people themselves are in control, and feel strengthened and uplifted by what they can achieve. The key to all we are talking about is what we have called the "bottom line" for PCHP, that is, *community control*. If this can work in the developing world where the weight of expert opinion would surely be that it could not succeed, how much more could such an approach work in the developed world, where the barriers are theoretically not so formidable? At the same time, the fact that these projects are succeeding could be taken as a testimony to the power of community, which is generally more intact in the developing world.

However, the reality of much of the world, developed or developing, is as old as history and prehistory. That is, a few people like to aggregate power and resources into their own hands, largely through motives of greed, fear, aggression, power and self-interest, and then use the rest of the population to suit their purposes. This does not take a single form, of course, and it can be in different grades of intensity, ranging from whole tyrannized nations, to the more subtle corporate and political controls in "developed" countries.

Because the most powerful are "in control", their values are the ones that most nations and communities are run by—that is, by the power of physical or material advantage, rather than by "moral" or "earned" power. We tend to accept this as the norm—that human existence is controlled by physical and material power, rather than by other "softer" values, such as consideration for others, respect, dignity, a sense of community, fairness, honouring the weak, and so on. Yet our experience from community work is that the *majority* of people, regardless of culture, class, gender, age or any other factor, are basically "decent" and want a society and a life for themselves and others that is much closer to these "soft" values than to the "hard" values of those who have the political and material power.

Somehow, the political lords and masters, and the big controlling corporations, running as they do by their own agendas, do not capture the hearts of the majority. So why is it that the "softer" values do not have a more influential voice in our societies? Partly it may be because there is no unified expression of these values that most of us share. But also, partly, it may be that we think others share the exploitative values of the minority who are in power—whereas our claim is that the opposite is true. That is, more people share the "soft" values. So how is it possible to articulate these "soft" values in a cohesive way in a society?

The first step may be to set up, both within nations and internationally, organizations that can articulate these values in a united way. These are the "good" and "noble" values that most cultures of all time have largely been in agreement about.

The next step would be to provide mechanisms at the *local* level to allow people to articulate, in terms of their own living situations, their individual and collective aspirations and wishes, in much the same way as we have described for the People System in this book. The process of collecting that information, and collating it at the local level to get a set of agreed-on priorities, is actually reasonably simple. It is just that no one does it. Then, having done this, one would aggregate local priorities into larger bundles, so that regional and national values, wishes and priorities could be known. The principle here is that this is driven from the periphery, from the local community level, whereas almost all government and social policy-making from the beginning of time, in all settings, has been driven from the centre— from those born or elected to govern, or, failing that, from those who force their way into positions of governing. No democracy is a true democracy— we elect governments to be autocracies for three to five years, and they then think they know what is best for us. And, often, they are wrong, as the huge dissatisfaction with electoral processes all over the world currently shows. What is the solution? Just what we are saying. To set up ongoing processes starting at the periphery, at the local community level, to gather information, and then to aggregate that information so that it finally ends up at the centre—rather than having the centre do it all.

This is not an argument for anarchy, which is a criticism some make of this kind of approach. We have seen that, in PCHP, the very essence is good organization. We see exactly the same being the case here. Another import- ant dimension is accepting that it all takes time—the information-gathering and collating, and the getting of agreement on priorities, have to be re- garded as requiring, perhaps, several years. But, once you have spent that time, the power of the information is so great that a strong base is built for the right action. You might say that the slowness of the process makes the information out of date before it is usable. We have never found this to be the case. The essentials never really change. If we have been waiting since the beginning of prehistory to get it right, what is wrong with a few more years?

To return to the PCHP perspective, we see that the action that would flow from a national priority-setting exercise would then come back to local communities. They would take their own local needs-assessment informa- tion, and blend that with the national perspective. But since the bottom line is community control, "the system" would have to acknowledge constitu- tionally that the balance of power, and in particular the control of local activities, is in the hands of the local people, not central government. The pattern of societal resource distribution would then have to reflect this. However, this would be the matter on which we see our grand vision being least palatable to central governments. It seems endemic to governments, whether of the left, right or centre, to aggregate more and more power to themselves, to have their own and corporate interests more at heart than the interests of "the people", and to exercise more and more power over the resources, which, as aggrieved taxpayers constantly remind us, is "our money"! All governments, almost by definition, seem to have totalitarian impulses!

We are not, however, arguing that community control is absolute. It is an absolute principle, but in practice it would require a balance between local

nd central imperatives. The concept that best fits here is that of "part-
ership", an equal power-sharing, involving negotiation, between the centre
nd the periphery. And, by the "periphery", we mean local, small-scale
ommunity—of perhaps no more than 10 000 people. Certainly our work
vith PCHP shows that, even in mixed urban communities, it is possible over
ime to develop strong concepts of local community, and for people to grow
bassionate about the place they live in, when perhaps that was not the
eality before. This is on the assumption that almost everyone, deep down,
las a yearning to return to small-scale, supportive community, and to relate
o those physically around them in a positive way. (This is not decrying the
value of other "communities", such as work groups, issue-based groups, or
hose who keep in touch by the telephone or the Internet, but it is not those
ve are talking about here. We are talking about old-fashioned local com-
nunity, where the bond is sharing the same piece of land, even if one only
sleeps there at night!)

     Having decided on this as a general strategic way of going about things,
hen the next step is to get a consensus on values. Because the values we are
alking about here are "soft", as opposed to dollars and force, which are
'hard", it is difficult for politicians and the big corporations to get their
leads around their significance. But such values are what drive our lives.
Often they are not explicit, but they are there nevertheless. Values are essen-
ially those emotionally held beliefs that make us decide to do one thing as
opposed to another. And, if the "soft" values are not explicitly articulated,
hen the "hard" implicit values are bound to win by default—these hard
unspoken values being mainly to do with dominating others through
noney, force and violence.

     And, in spite of there being no single articulated set of values among
'ordinary people" (the jpf's!), there is no doubt to us, based on our past and
current community work, that there is a broad consensus on "soft" values
among the majority of people. These include such things as the desire to do
vell by one's children, the wish to contribute meaningfully to society, the
desire to have opportunities to get together with others at the community
evel, the wish to help those who are incapacitated or otherwise temporarily
or permanently at a disadvantage, the wish for respect and dignity to be
shown towards oneself and also to show that to others, the wish to be loved
or at least respected by others, the desire for a sense of community, the wish
for a pleasant community environment with good facilities, the desire to
acquire new knowledge and skills regardless of age, and the desire for a
'fair deal" for everyone. All these things and more come out in every survey
we have done, and we are always amazed by it. These shared values seem to
span all classes, all cultures and all age groups. We are not saying that every
single person in a community will have all these values, but collectively they
are there in the majority. And this is true even where the immediate

behaviour of someone would suggest the opposite. The parent who batters an infant is unlikely to have child-battering as a "value". Indeed, she or he probably has caring well for their children as a value. But circumstances stress, drugs and other such things drive many to engage in actions no necessarily consonant with their "real" values. However, if one takes a developmental perspective (that is, it takes time), this kind of situation is something that can be successfully tackled at the community level, as one sees in so many projects, and as individual and community strengths increase, so too does the capacity to express the "soft" values.

However, the sceptic may be in doubt about the prevalence of the "soft" values we are talking about here. After all, look at all the "bad news" we read about in the newspapers or see on television every day! Doesn't that mean that most people are awful? And look at all the bigotry and prejudice we hear expressed. However, we assert that one of the great tragedies of modern society is that most of us simply do not know what most other people really think or feel. Our information sources about this tend to be the media and the entertainment industry, and it would be hard to think of a more distorted set of sources than these! And then we have all developed multiple prejudices and opinions about people and groups as part of our culture, class and upbringing, and these are an even *worse* source of accurate information about the reality of other people. We submit that the only real source of good information about others is the sort of community values/ needs surveys and forums that we have discussed with regard to PCHP Sadly, these barely exist. Even "opinion surveys" are mostly shallow, and are usually driven by media, political or interest group imperatives. So the majority of us tend to go on in ignorance of the fact that 90% of other people are probably quite like us in their basic "soft" values, even though these take a variety of expressions, and may be hidden from time to time. Not a bad starting point is to assume that the majority of people are "good". But how many of us genuinely believe this? Of course, there are exceptions to this widespread "goodness", but in general we believe—know—it to be true. And, if you do not believe it, then do your own survey to check it out!

Now we would like to return to the PEOPLE analysis we presented at the beginning of this book, to summarize what we are talking about here.

P: People-centredness

As can be seen, at the heart of this "new society" is a powerful commitment to operating that society in terms of what the people feel deeply they want for themselves. The perspective for this is the opposite of the distorted, Olympian view of remote central governments, of politicians whose own lives are almost by definition "abnormal". Rather, the central perspective in this new society is the viewpoint of ordinary people nested in their everyday community lives, which is where the life of any society really happens. The task is then simply to seek, and make the basis of social and political action, a representative expression of what people really want for themselves at that level. What we hope we have shown with this book is that that process is not just an ideal—it can quite readily be done.

E: Empowerment

This is the number one value, of course. You might feel like saying to us: "Aren't *you* imposing *your* values on others?" In particular, you might ask: "*Do* people actually *want* to be empowered? Don't they want others to make decisions for them?" Our reply to that is: "Check it out with the people!" Our overwhelming impression from years of community work is that what the vast majority of ordinary people want for themselves and their communities is exactly what we have been trying to communicate in this book. Especially, they want what we have tried to represent by the term "empowerment". That is, virtually everyone wants to make decisions about, and to have control over, his or her life, to have maximal opportunity for self-determination, and to develop knowledge, strengths and skills according to one's own agendas. Most also acknowledge that there is tremendous value in local collective efforts for making a better community and society. Obviously, not everyone wants to be actively involved in community activities. However, we do find a remarkable percentage who do want to be, and what is absent is not their motivation, but the opportunity, facilities and organizational structures for them to be able to do this.

O: Organizational and Community Development

As we say, what we are talking about here is emphatically not anarchy. The whole process is one that is orderly and somewhat slow. The requisite management and organizational systems are carefully thought out, and actions are matched to available resources. The evaluative component is also crucial in this. What is involved are organic changes in communities (and societies), with the majority of people participating, and which take place at a rate required to ensure that there is stability, certainty and belief in what is going on. What would be needed here for this to take place at a societal level are government policies (centrally set up, we must say!) and cultural frameworks that would make all this happen. These would be required to protect the "soft" and fragile processes involved from the "forces of evil", which not only include sabotage from those who do not like what is going on, but also include "reversion to type" if one is not aware constantly of the goals and the organizational imperatives. In this approach, the most basic "unit" at the societal level is "the community", and "community development" is the central strategy.

P: Participation

The real strength behind community-based action is participation. As we discussed earlier, participation is the principal vehicle for empowerment at the community level. Also, our surveys tend to suggest that "participation" in some form is perhaps the number one wish of people at the community level. (Note: As well as politicians, we find many academics do not like this kind of view, because by their nature they tend to be neither participatory nor "community people". Heaven forbid that our society be run by academics!) Because in advocating this approach we are faced with the likely opposition of governments, the corporate sector, academics and other such vested interests, we need our power base to be as strong as possible. This power base comes through participation—through large numbers of ordinary people united in a common certainty that what we are talking about here is the "best way". Our surveys show without doubt that the majority of ordinary people *do* think that way, but there is a big step between having that knowledge, and setting up the community and social structures required to enact that way of societal functioning. The only way that will happen is through "people power", and people power means constructive participation and united purpose, through people sharing in activities considered to be of social value both to oneself and to others. As we have seen, substantial, indeed majority, participation can be achieved through the kind of locality- and wishes-based approach we have presented in this book. Such participation is the key to success in this venture, and also the key to a satisfying life for the majority of people.

L: Life Quality

It should be clear that the overriding goal of what we are advocating here is subjectively experienced quality of life of the type we discussed in Chapter 4. And here, we have to emphasize the *equity* aspect of this. What we are talking about here is quality of life for *everyone*. It is beyond the scope of this discussion to go into detail about this, but our concept is one of "Basic quality of life". "Basic quality of life" is a "lower limit" criterion of quality for life for which there is a social and political consensus, and agreement about its status as a basic human necessity for everyone in a society. "Basic quality of life" would combine two broad sectors, one being the obvious external factors such as income, opportunity for work, access to societal resources and services, and a pleasant living environment, and the other being more subtle psychological or "empowerment" factors such as school programmes that enhance self-esteem and strength-building, workplace philosophies that support this approach, honouring culture, making special efforts for those who normally do not get heard or get overlooked, encouraging parenting skills and good facilities for preschoolers, neighbourhood development programmes, and so on. This latter, more "subtle" sector would involve factors that were more "programmatic" than "structural" (although facilities would be an important part of this sector). And, of course, any programmes and facilities would be decided on, and controlled by, local people. As we say, the equity dimension is uppermost here. This is not to say we are advocating the same quality of life for everyone. Rather, the aim is to have *a basic level of quality of life* agreed on by, and regarded as a necessity for, everyone in a society. It is envisaged that this basic level would need to be well above the only "life quality indicator" most developed countries have at present—"the poverty line"—and it obviously is much more complex than just minimum income. Some people may want to throw up their hands in horror at the thought of trying to figure out what this mix of requirements would be, and at what level. But we would like to suggest a simple principle here—that of common sense and goodwill. Anybody with a bit of sense and goodwill can judge whether a situation is okay or not in terms of quality of life, and that is what we are talking about here. This is not a do-gooder ethic, or saying that we have to structure society for the good of others on a "we know what is best for people" basis (which has sometimes been the approach of conventional health promotion). On the contrary, we are committed, as must be clear, to people deciding for themselves what is good for them, within a knowledge of resource constraints. And, if a society is committed to this sort of approach, those resource constraints may be less than one might think. Obviously, "equity" issues involve public resource distribution issues. But again we argue the need for simple "common sense/goodwill" judgements, rather than trying to work out hard and fast mathematical formulae. We are talking about *intention*—and to quote that cliché again: where there is a will, there is a way!

Giving a primary role to experienced life quality in our society would have a lot of repercussions. It would mean respecting culture and the deepest parts of the human spirit. It would mean giving time to the softer dimension of life—the beauty, the joy, the gentleness, the nobility of humankind. It means taking into account all dimensions of life, beyond "health", or even "mental health", to the whole of existence.

Quality of life, then, is our focus and goal, and that means not only for everyone in our own society, but for every single person on this planet.

E: Evaluation

As must be quite clear to every reader of this book, we favour an evaluative organizational system based on clearly specified goals, with constant monitoring of progress toward their attainment. These requirements would be crucial if we are to move towards the kind of sociopolitical environment we are talking about here. Goals, based on the collective wishes of communities, would be clearly known and decided on consensually—a process we have demonstrated is relatively easy to do. All activities would be evaluated in terms of their moving toward the attainment of goals on a cybernetics or self-optimizing model. Other evaluative information, both quantitative and qualitative, would be needed to supplement goal-attainment data, to ensure that the processes are working as well as possible, that people are satisfied with what is happening, that quality of life is indeed being affected positively, and that all sectors of society are being included on an equitable basis. Continual needs-assessment processes would have to be part of this too.

Before we end, we should also mention in this context the two "new" concepts this book introduced to the health promotion discourse—culture and spirituality. Any agenda of the type we are talking about here would need to be very cognizant of these. Many indigenous world cultures are currently at risk, and since, like community, people's essential identity and place in the world is inextricably tied up with their culture, then it is vital that respect for culture be put right up front as a central societal value.

And then there is the "softest" value of all—that of spirituality. Given a world dominated by "hard" values, it is no wonder that, in many modern societies, spirituality and religion are in disarray. But, again, the reality (as determined from research) seems different from the popular stereotypes. For example, in New Zealand, the census shows that only about 10% of people report they go to church or engage in formal religious observance. However, other research shows that 70% of the population believe in "something", or have a spiritual leaning. Therefore, there is a substantial gap between what society currently "provides" to meet people's spiritual needs, and what appear to be the overall interests in this area. Of course, keeping private about one's spirituality may be the wish of most of these people. However, our sense from our community work is not only that there is a strong and widespread interest in "spirituality" broadly defined, but also that many people would like some community-based opportunity for its expression. However, at present, not even "good" community projects seem to address this issue systematically (beyond those linked with specific religions). Furthermore, discussion of this area does not even appear to be on the health promotion agenda—usually regarded as being avant-garde in its social concerns—much less any other social or political agenda. Spirituality represents our relationship to the profoundest aspects of individual and collective human existence and, we believe, any vision for a new society must take this dimension into account.

To sum up, then, we think the "vision" we have presented here is eminently feasible. We believe we have shown in this book that its essential elements can be implemented in a relatively straightforward way at the community level and, to some extent, at the regional and national level. But the book only does this for that sector of activity called "health promotion". Not only is that a very small part of even the most developed country's public activities, but it may well be a dying enterprise, given the monetarist-driven restructuring that has been taking place in many modern health systems. To the extent that the "hard" values triumph in a society, the "soft" values of health promotion, and the kind of vision we have given here, are likely to fade even further off the public agenda.

This is, of course, no reason to give up on this sort of "visioning". And we firmly believe that, given a world that psychologically gets smaller by the year, it is not enough just to do this "visioning" at a national level. This book, written by two people living at opposite ends of the earth, is a good example of this shrinking world. We share the same basic values, and know that many others, if not the majority of other people around the world, share broadly the same values. So what we also need is an *international* vision— not one that is imposed by us or anyone else, but one that emerges from the kind of participatory, consultative, empowering approach we advocate here. We see some promising signs in this direction. For example, there are influential national bodies that are starting to address such questions as: What is a fair society? At an international level, the United Nations Human Development Index is also a start in this direction. We would see the latter as a first step towards an international consensus on what constitutes basic quality of life for everyone in the world. The universal availability of the Internet and its potential to link up people of good heart around the world is also a vital component of this. We sometimes hear that the world is being run by a cartel of international financiers who exist behind closed doors in various capitals of the world, and manipulate the global economy to their advantage. This may or may not be true. But, if the world is being run by such a group, then the need for an international effort of the kind we are talking about here is even more vital. It is easy to be pessimistic about the enormity of the task. But when one sees what the grass-roots groups we mentioned above have achieved, and likewise thousands of other wonderful community-based projects and movements around the world, then in spite of what seems like the most absurd odds, we are sure it can be done. What is needed is the shared vision, and the will and the organizational structures, to set it up. What is needed is participation, a people orientation, and empowerment. So how about it, dear reader?

REFERENCES

Adams, M. (1993) Report to Roy McKenzie Foundation on the Cairns Workshop on Social Change, Community Empowerment and Enablement, Cairns, Australia, 2–9 October 1993. Unpublished document.

Alinsky, S. D. (1972) *Rules for Radicals*. New York: Random House.

Antonovsky, A. (1979) *Health, Stress and Coping*. San Francisco: Jossey-Bass.

Antonovsky, A. (1987) *Unravelling the Mystery of Health: How People Manage Stress and Stay Well*. San Francisco, CA: Jossey-Bass.

Ariyaratne, A. T. (1985) *Collected Works*, vol. III. Sri Lanka: Sarvodaya Shramadana.

Arnstein, S. (1969) A ladder of citizen participation. *AIP Journal*, July, 216.

Auckland Star (1982) Happiness is Birkenhead, St Heliers: Auckland Research Group/Auckland Star Survey. *Auckland Star*, 31 August, 1–3.

Bandura, A. (1977) Self-efficacy: Toward a unifying theory of behavioral change. *Psychological Review*, **84**, 91–215.

Battisti, T. (1995) *Rapid assessment methods in community health development*. Unpublished Master of Public Health thesis, University of Auckland.

Benson, H. (1975) *The Relaxation Response*. London: Collins.

Bethwaite, P., Baker, M., Pearce, N. and Kawachi, I. (1990) Unemployment and the public health. *New Zealand Medical Journal*, **103**, 48–49.

Bivins, E. C. (1979) Community organization—an old but reliable health education technique. In P. M. Lazes (Ed.), *The Handbook of Health Education*, pp. 109–130. Germantown, MD: Aspen.

Bourguignon, E. (Ed.) (1973) Introduction. In *Religion, Altered States of Consciousness, and Social Change*. Columbus, OH: Ohio State University Press.

Boyte, H. C. (1989) People power transforms a St Louis housing project. *Utne Reader*, **34**, 46–47.

Brandon, D. (1976) *Zen in the Art of Helping*. London: Routledge & Kegan-Paul.

Breckon, D. J., Harvey, J. R. and Lancaster, R. B. (1985) *Community Health Education*. Rockville, MD: Aspen.

Bridgman, G. (1993) Maori at risk. In H. Williams (Ed.), *Why the Treaty of Waitangi is Important*. Auckland: Mental Health Foundation of New Zealand.

Brown, P., Galan, M. and Henley, N. (1974) *The Radical Therapist*. Harmondsworth: Penguin.

Callahan, D. (1990) *What Kind of Life: The Limits of Medical Progress*. New York: Simon & Schuster.

Capra, F. (1987) *The Tao of Physics*. Bungay, UK: Fontana.

Churchman, C. W. (1968) *The Systems Approach*. New York: Delta.

Claxton, G. (1986) *Beyond Therapy: The Impact of Eastern Religions on Psychological Theory and Practice*. London: Wisdom.

Cohen, F. and Lazarus, R. (1983) Coping and adaptation in health and illness. In D. Mechanic (Ed.), *Handbook of Health, Health Care, and the Health Professions*. New York: Free Press.

Cohen, J. M. and Phipps, J.-F. *The Common Experience*. London: Rider.

Cohen, S. and Syme, S. L. (Eds) (1985) *Social Support and Health*. New York: Academic Press.

Delbecq, A., Van De Ven, A. H. and Gustafson, D. H. (1975) *Group Techniques for Programme Planning: A Guide to Nominal Group and Delphi Processes*. Glenview, IL: Dorsey Press.

Dignan, M. H. and Carr, P. C. (1981) *Introduction to Program Planning: A Basic Text for Community Health Education*. Philadelphia, PA: Lea & Febiger.

Durning, A. B. (1989) Grass roots groups are our best hope for global prosperity and ecology. *Utne Reader*, **34**, 40–49.

Ellis, A. and Grieger, R. (Eds) (1977) *Handbook of Rational–Emotive Therapy*. New York: Springer.

Epp, J. (1986) *Achieving Health for All: A Framework for Health Promotion*. Ottawa: Health & Welfare Canada.

Feldman, R. E. (1979) Collaborative consultation: A process for joint professional–consumer development of primary prevention programs. *Journal of Community Psychology*, **7**, 118–128.

Fellin, P. (1987) *The Competent Community*. Itasca, IL: Peacock.

Feng, G.-F. and English, J. (1972) *Tao Te Ching*. London: Wildwood House.

Foreyt, J. P. and Kondo, A. T. (1984) Advances in behavioral treatment of obesity. In M. Herson and R. M. Esler (Eds), *Progress in Behavior Modification*, vol. 16. Orlando, FL: Academic Press.

Freire, P. (1972) *Pedagogy of the Oppressed*. Harmondsworth: Penguin.

Freyssinet, J. (1966) *Le Concept de Sous-Developpement*. Paris: Mouton.

Garvin, C. D. and Cox, F. M. (1987) A history of community organizing since the civil war with special reference to oppressed communities. *Strategies of Community Organizing*. (4th edn). Englewood Cliffs, NJ: Prentice-Hall.

Goswami, A. (1993) *The Self-Aware Universe: How Consciousness Creates the Material World*. New York: Tarcher/Putnam.

Grace, V. (1991) *Orienting health promotion practice*. Papers from the Health Promotion Forum First National Conference. Auckland: Health Promotion Forum of New Zealand.

Homans, G. (1950) *The Small Group*. New York: Harcourt.

Hope, A. and Timmel, S. (1984) *Training for Transformation: A Handbook for Community Workers*. Gwern, Zimbabwe: Mambo Press.

Howlett, M. and Archer, V. (1984) Worker involvement in occupational health and safety. *Family and Community Health*, November, 57–63.

Huxley, A. (1961) *The Perennial Philosophy*. London: Fontana.

Huxley, A. (1962) Introduction. In S. Prabhavananda and C. Isherwood (Eds), *The Song of God: Bhagavad-Gita*. New York: Mentor.

Israel, B. (1985) Social networks and social support: Implications for natural helpers and community level interventions. *Health Education Quarterly*, **12**, 66–80.

James, W (1902) *The Varieties of Religious Experience: A Study in Human Nature*, 1961 edn. New York: Collier.

Kapleau, P. (1965) *The Three Pillars of Zen*. Boston, MA: Beacon Press.

Khoshkhoo, A. G. (1996) *Community development, unemployment and health: Initial research for the Other Way Project in Northcote*. Unpublished Master of Health Science thesis, University of Auckland.

Kieffer, C. (1984) Citizen empowerment: A developmental perspective. *Prevention in Human Services*, **3**, 9–36.

Kinloch, P. (1985) *Talking Health but Doing Sickness: Studies in Samoan Health*. Wellington: Victoria University Press.

Kobasa, S. C. O., Maddi, S. R., Pucetti, M. C. and Zola, M. A. (1985) Effectiveness of hardiness, exercise and social support as resources against illness. *Journal of Psychosomatic Research*, **29**, 525–533.

Labonte, R. (1990) Empowerment: Notes on community and professional dimensions. *Canadian Research on Social Policy*, **26**, 64–75.

Labonte, R. (1993) Health promotion and empowerment: Practice frameworks. *Issues in Health Promotion*, vol. III. Toronto: Centre for Health Promotion/ ParticipACTION.

Lalonde, M. (1974) *A New Perspective on the Health of Canadians*. Ottawa: Information Canada.

Lave, J. (1988) *Cognition in Practice: Mind, Mathematics and Practice in Everyday Life*. New York: Cambridge University Press.

Little Bear, L., Boldt, M. and Long, J. A. (1984) *Pathways to Self-Determination: Canadian Indians and the Canadian State*. Toronto: University of Toronto Press.

Locke, S., Ader, R., Besedovsky, H., Hall, N., Solomon, G. and Strom, T. (Eds) (1985) *Foundations of Psychoneuroimmunology*. New York: Aldine.

Lord, J. and Farlow, D. M. (1990) A study of personal empowerment: Implications for health promotion. *Health Promotion (Canada)*, **29**, 2–8.

Lynch, J. J. (1977) *The Broken Heart: The Medical Consequences of Loneliness*. New York: Basic Books.

McCreary, J. and Shirley, I. (1982) In the rural tradition: Anthropologists come to town. In I. Shirley (Ed.), *Development Tracks: The Theory and Practice of Community Development*. Palmerston North: Dunmore Press.

McCullum. H. and McCullum, K. (1975) *This Land is Not for Sale*. Toronto: Anglican Book Centre.

Maclean, H. M. and Eakin, J. M. (Eds) (1992) Health promotion research methods: Expanding the repertoire. *Canadian Journal of Public Health*, Suppl. 1, 83.

McLeod, B. (1986) Prescription for health: A dose of self-confidence. *Psychology Today*, October, 46–50.

Marsden, M. (1992) God, man and universe: A Maori view. In M. King (Ed.), *Te Ao Hurihuri: Aspects of Maoritanga*. Auckland: Reed.

Maslow, A. (1973) *The Further Reaches of Human Nature*. Harmondsworth: Penguin.

Maynard, J. and Merhten, J. (1995) The fourth wave: A new paradigm for business. *The Systems Thinker*, **6**, 9–11.

Metge, J. and Kinloch, P. (1978) *Talking Past Each Other: Problems of Cross-Cultural Communication*. Wellington: Victoria University Press and Price Milburn.

Miller, M. (1985) Turning problems into actionable issues. Unpublished report, Organize Training Center, San Francisco.

Minkler, M. (1990) Improving health through community organization. In K. Glanz, F. M. Lewis and B. K. Rimer (Eds), *Health Behavior and Health Education*, pp. 257–287. San Francisco, CA: Jossey-Bass.

Mowat, C. L. (1961) *The Charity Organization Society, 1869–1913*. London: Methuen.

Neher, A. (1980) *The Psychology of Transcendence*. Englewood Cliffs, NJ: Prentice-Hall.

Ngan-Woo, F. (1990) *Faasamoa: The World of Samoans*. Auckland: Office of the Race Relations Conciliator.

Nhat Hanh, T. (1987) *Being Peace*. Berkeley, CA: Parallax Press.

North Shore Times Advertizer (1979) "Best community project in NZ" gets $5500. *North Shore Times Advertizer*, 24 May, 3.

Ottawa Charter for Health Promotion (1986) *Health Promotion*, **1**, iii–v.

Patel, C. (1993) Mental health (among Maori). In H. Williams (Ed.), *Why the Treaty of Waitangi is Important*. Auckland: Mental Health Foundation of New Zealand.

Pransky, J. (1991) *Prevention: The Critical Need.* Springfield, MO: Burrell Foundation.

Raeburn, J. M. (1976) Community Push: A community-oriented evaluation programme in a psychiatric ward. *Australian and New Zealand Journal of Psychiatry*, **10**, 305–310.

Raeburn, J. M. (1985) Expressed interest in health-related lifestyle change in three communities. *New Zealand Medical Journal*, **98**, 242–244.

Raeburn, J. M. (1987) People projects: Planning and evaluation in a new era. *Health Promotion (Canada)*, **25**, 2–13.

Raeburn, J. M. (1992) *The Other Way Project.* University of Auckland. Unpublished document.

Raeburn, J. M. and Atkinson, J. E. (1986) A low-cost community approach to weight control: Initial results from an evaluated trial. *Preventive Medicine*, **15**, 391–402.

Raeburn, J. M. and Seymour, F. W. (1979) A simple systems model for community programs. *Journal of Community Psychology*, **7**, 290–297.

Raeburn, J. M., Atkinson, J. E., Dubignon, J. M., McPherson, M. and Elkind, G. S. (1993) "Unstress": A low-cost community psychology approach to stress-management: An evaluated case study from New Zealand. *Journal of Community Psychology*, **21**, 113–123.

Raeburn, J. M., Atkinson, J. E., Dubignon, J. M., Fitzpatrick, J., McPherson, M. and Elkind, G. (1994) Superhealth Basic: Development and evaluation of a low-cost community-based lifestyle programme. *Psychology and Health*, **9**, 383–395.

Rangihau, J. (1992) Being Maori. In M. King (Ed.), *Te Ao Hurihuri: Aspects of Maoritanga.* Auckland: Reed.

Rappaport, J. (1981) In praise of paradox: A social policy of empowerment over prevention. *American Journal of Community Psychology*, **9**, 1–25.

Rappaport, J. (1984) Studies in empowerment: Introduction to the issue. *Prevention in Human Services*, **3**, 1–7.

Rappaport, J. (1987) Terms of empowerment/exemplars of prevention: Towards a theory for community psychology. *Journal of Community Psychology*, **15**, 2.

Rappaport, J. (1992) Research methods and the empowerment social agenda. In P. Tolan, C. Keys, F. Chertok and L. Jason (Eds) *Researching Community Psychology.* Washington, DC: American Psychological Association.

Rissel, C. (1994) Empowerment: The holy grail of health promotion? *Health Promotional International*, **9**, 39–47.

Robertson, A. and Minkler, M. (1994) New health promotion movement: A critical examination. *Health Education Quarterly*, **21**, 295–312.

Ross, M. (1955) *Community Organization: Theory and Principles.* New York: Harper & Row.

Ross, M. (1967) *Community Organization: Theory, Principles and Practice.* New York: Harper & Row.

Rothman, J. and Tropman, J. E. (1987) Models of community organization and macro practice perspectives: Their mixing and phasing. In F. M. Cox, J. L. Erlich, J. Rothman and J. E. Tropman (Eds), *Strategies of Community Organization: Macro-Practice*, 4th edn. Itasca, IL: Peacock.

Sampson, E. E. (1991) The democratization of psychology. *Theory and Psychology*, **1**, 275–298.

Sarafino, E. P. (1994) *Health Psychology: Biopsychosocial Interactions*, 2nd edn. New York: Wiley.

Sarason, S. B. (1974) *The Psychological Sense of Community: Prospects for a Community Psychology.* San Francisco, CA: Jossey-Bass.

Schloegl, I. (1975) *The Wisdom of the Zen Masters.* London: Sheldon Press.

Seedhouse, D. (1988) *Ethics: The Heart of Health Care.* Chichester: Wiley.

Seers, D. (1972) What are we trying to measure? In N. Baster (Ed.), *Measuring Development*. Frank Cass.

Senge, P. M. (1994) *The Fifth Discipline: The Art and Practice of the Learning Organization*, 2nd edn. New York: Currency Doubleday.

Sherif, M. (1966) *In Common Predicament: The Social Psychology of Intergroup Conflict and Cooperation*. Boston, MA: Houghton-Mifflin.

Shirley, I. (Ed.) (1982) *Development Tracks: The Theory and Practice of Community Development*. Palmerston North: Dunmore Press.

Spreitzer, G. (1995) An empirical test of a comprehensive model of intrapersonal empowerment in the workplace. *American Journal of Community Psychology*, **23**, 6001–6029.

Steptoe, A. and Appels, A. (1989) *Stress, Personal Control and Health*. Chichester: Wiley.

Stuart, R. B. (1967) Behavioral control of overeating. *Behavior Research and Therapy*, **5**, 357–365.

Stunkard, A. J. and Penick, S. B. (1982) Obesity. In A. S. Bellack, M. Hersen and A. E. Kazdin (Eds), *International Handbook of Behavior Modification and Therapy*. New York: Plenum.

Surgeon General (1979) *Healthy people: The Surgeon General's report on health promotion and disease prevention*. Washington, DC: US Government.

Syme, S. L. (1989) Control and health: a personal perspective. In A. Steptoe and A. Appels (Eds), *Stress, Personal Control and Health*. Chichester: Wiley.

Thackeray, M. G., Skidmore, R. A. and Farley, O. W. (1979) *Introduction to Mental Health: Field and Practice*. Englewood Cliffs, NJ: Prentice-Hall.

Trungpa, C. (1973) *Cutting Through Spiritual Materialism*. Stuart & Watkins.

Van de Ven, A. H. and Poole, M. S. (1995) Explaining development and change in organizations. *Academy of Management Review*, **20**, 510–540.

von Bertalanffy, L. (1968) *General System Theory*. Harmondsworth: Penguin.

Walker, R. (1982) Development from below: Institutional transformation in a plural society. In I. Shirley (Ed.), *Development Tracks: The Theory and Practice of Community Development*. Palmerston North: Dunmore Press.

Wallerstein, N. (1992) Powerlessness, empowerment and health: Implications for health promotion programs. *American Journal of Health Promotion*, **6**, 197–205.

Walsh, R. N. and Vaughan, F. E. (Eds) (1993) *Paths Beyond Ego: The Transpersonal Vision*. Los Angeles, CA: Tarcher/Perigree.

Watts, A. (1975) *Tao: The Watercourse Way*. New York: Pantheon.

Weber, M. (1946) Science as a vocation. In H. H. Garth and C. W. Mills (Eds), *Max Weber: Essays in Sociology*. Oxford University Press.

Weissman, H. (1982) Fantasy and reality of staff involvement in organizational change. *Administration in Social Work*, **6**, 37–45.

Williams, H. (1993) Treaty of Waitangi summary. In H. Williams (Ed.), *Why the Treaty of Waitangi is Important*. Auckland: Mental Health Foundation of New Zealand.

Woodill, G., Renwick, R., Brown, I. and Raphael, D. (1994) Being, belonging, becoming: An approach to the quality of life in persons with developmental disabilities. In D. Goode (Ed.), *Quality of Life for Persons with Developmental Disabilities: International Perspectives and Issues*, pp. 57–74. Cambridge, MA: Brookline.

Zukav, G. (1979) *The Dancing Wu-Li Masters: An Overview of the New Physics*. Bungay, UK: Fontana.

INDEX

accountability   42, 153
activities, participation in   32–3
  empowerment   66–7
Alma Ata Declaration (1978)   89

behaviour modification   5
biopsychosocial model of health   12–14
Birkdale–Beachhaven Community
  Project   172–81

Canada
  cultures   99–100
    native Canadians   108–9
  Lalonde Report   3–4
  Ontario Disability Project   53–5
  Workplace Health System   27–8
cardiovascular health, psychological
  factors   13
care, personal, empowerment   74–5
choice, quality of life   55
coalitions, empowerment   75–6
community   10
  delineation   89–90, 133
  diversity in   29–30
  strength-building within   24
  transpersonal self and   119–21
  unity   33–4
community action, spirituality
    and   121–5
community activities   32–3
  empowerment   66–7
community control   10–11, 22, 214–16
  developing countries   92–7
community development   26, 28–9,
    80–97
  developing countries   92–7
  empowerment   86–8, 91
  health education model   84–92

    historical/conceptual
      dimensions   81–4
    ideal society   219
    organizational development and
      26–8
  community of interest (COI)   139
  community organization   84–92
    empowerment   75
  community perspective   18–19
  community psychology   14, 48
    view of empowerment   67–9
  Community Push programme   168,
    169–72
  compassion   122
  competence
    community   91
    participatory   71–3, 77–8
  conscientization, community
    organization   92
  consultation, PCHP project   139–40,
    141, 143
  control
    community   10–11, 22, 214–16
      developing countries   92–7
    group   23
    personal   12, 23, 24, 65
    political and material   215–16
    quality of life   55
    research   162–3
  crisis situations   48
  culture
    health and   98–110
      experiential perspective   99–104
      Maoris   104–8
      native Canadians   108–9
      pressure to change   101
    ideal society   222
  cybernetics   41–2, 136

data
  experiential (subjective)   16–18
  objective indices   40, 157–8
  ownership   42–3
  participation statistics   155–6
  power   43
dependency   25
development
  community *see* community
        development
  as concept   80–1
  in empowerment   70–3
  organizational   26–8
    ideal society   219
disability, Ontario Project   53–5

Eatwell programme   191–3
ecological approach   132–3
education
  community development and   82–3
  health *see* health education
ego, phenomenal   117, 119
employees, empowerment   27
Empowering Resource Centre
      (ERC)   198
empowerment   11, 21–6, 64–79
  community development   86–8, 91
  community psychology view   67–9
  ideal society   219
  leadership skills   141
  mentor   66, 77
  in PCHP   76–9
  personal   12
    developmental perspective   70–3
    experiential   64–7, 70–3
  philosophy/ideology   69
  practical application   130–1
  psychological components   73
  social factors   66
  structural perspective   73–6
Empowerment Holosphere
      (Labonte)   74–6
errors   136
evaluation   39–43, 133–4
  cybernetics   41–2, 136
  ideal society   221–2
  outcome *see* outcome evaluation
  process   40–1
experiential data   16–18

feedback, cybernetics   41–2, 136

funding   147

General System Theory   135
generic approach   132–3
goals   35, 45, 133–4
  attainment
    evaluation   39–40, 154–5
    subprojects for   148–9
  People System   136
  review   41, 149–50
  setting   143–4, 149
    goal-setting and review
        meetings   149–50
  ultimate   35–6
groups
  control   23
  empowerment   75, 77
  participation and   30–1
  strength-building within   24
  target   31, 133

health
  health promotion context   9–10
  and quality of life   59–60
  subjective measures   40, 158–60
  WHO definition   8, 56, 59
health education, community
      development and   84–92
Health Field Concept, Lalonde
      Report   4
health promotion
  agents   10–11
  description/definition   8–11
  history   3–7
  quality of life and   60–3
holistic approach   132–3

ill-being   36, 56–63
immune system, psychological
      factors   13
Impact Questionnaire   158–60
incorporated society   131, 144–5
  Birkdale–Beachhaven Community
        Project   174
individual, role in health promotion   7
issue selection, community
      organization   92

Lalonde Report   3–4
land
  Maori culture   104–8

native Canadian culture   108, 109
leadership development   91, 140
learning organizations   27
lifestyle
   Lalonde Report   4
   social factors in   6
   Superhealth programmes   184–95
locality development, community
   organization   90

Maori culture   99
   community   107
   health and   106–7
   power of land   104–8
   subjectivity and   113
media   141
mental health
   Community Push programme   168,
     169–72
   North Shore Community Health
     Network   196, 197–203
mental models   27

needs assessment   131, 133–4
   Birkdale–Beachhaven Community
     Project   173–5
   People System   142–3
New Zealand
   Birkdale–Beachhaven Community
     Project   172–81
   Community Push programme   168,
     169–72
   cultures   99
   see also Maori culture
   North Shore Community Health
     Network   196, 197–203
   Other Way Project   196, 203–13
   Superhealth programme   182–95
North Shore Community Health
   Network   196, 197–203
nutrition, Eatwell programme   191–3

Ontario Disability Project   53–5
organization
   community   75, 84–92
   learning   27
organizational development (OD)   26–8
   ideal society   219
Other Way Project   196, 203–13
Ottawa Charter   6–7
outcome evaluation   39–40, 152–4

People System   152–66
   summary statement   164–5

participation   29–34
   community development/
     organization   83, 91
   empowerment   66–7, 71–3, 77–8
   ideal society   220
   statistics   155–6
people power   220
People System   134–7, 167–8
   Birkdale–Beachhaven Community
     Project   172–81
   Community Push programme   168,
     169–72
   North Shore Community Health
     Network   196, 197–203
   Other Way Project   196, 203–13
   outcome evaluation   152–66
     summary statement   164–5
   procedural steps   138–51
     goal-setting   143–4
     goal-setting and review
       meetings   149–50
     guidelines   150–1
     initial consultation   138–40
     initial organization   140–1
     needs assessment   142–3
     permanent organizational
       structure   144–5
     prioritization of needs   143–4
     re-examination of philosophy and
       objectives   145–6
     relationship between committee/
       board and staff   146–7
     resource planning   147
     subprojects   148–9
     worker requirements and
       guidelines   148
   Superhealth programme   182–95
people-centred health promotion
   (PCHP)
   key essentials   16–44
   principles   15
   application   129–37
   society based on   214–23
   projects see People System
   theoretical and political context   45–9
   ultimate goal   35–6
people-centredness   16–21
   ideal society   218–19

Perennial Philosophy   115–18
personal control   12, 23, 24, 65
personal mastery   27
phenomenal ego   117, 119
politics
  control and   215–16
  health promotion   45–8, 49
    community development   82–3
    empowerment   76, 77
positivism   17, 19
positivity   36–8
power   73–4, 78
  people   220
  political and material   215–16
  transpersonal and   118–19
  see also empowerment
prevention of disease   9, 35, 68
prioritization of needs   143–4
professionals
  facilitatory role   19–21, 25
  superior attitude   19–20
psychology
  as base for PCHP   17–18, 48
  community   14, 48
    view of empowerment   67–9
  health   12–14
  transpersonal   112
psychoneuroimmunology   13
publicity   141

qualitative studies   40, 161–2
quality of life (QOL)   35–8
  basic   220–1
  determinants   36, 56–63
  feedback loop   56, 57
  health and   59–60
  health promotion and   60, 62–3
  ideal society   220–1
  moderating conditions   56, 58, 60
  Ontario Disability Project   53–5
questionnaires, self-report   158–61

random survey
  needs assessment   142
  outcome evaluation   157
representativeness   31
research
  experiential   16–18
  ownership   42–3
  qualitative   40, 161–2

quasi-experimental, outcome
  evaluation   162–4
resources
  PCHP projects   147
  provision to community   25

Samoan (Western) culture   101, 102–4,
  117
satisfaction measures   40, 161
self   111–13, 119–21
  community and   119–21
  eternal   117
  non-ego   121–2
self-criticism   41
shared vision   27
social action, spirituality and
  121–5
social change, community
  organization   91
social model of health   6
  Ottawa Charter   6
social network techniques   91
social planning, community
  organization   90
social support   12–14
spirituality   38, 111–25
  ideal society   222
  Perennial Philosophy   115–18
  in social and community action
    121–5
statistics
  objective indices   40, 157–8
  participation   155–6
  power of   43
strength-building   12–14, 24
  practical application   132
stress management, Superhealth
  programme   186–9
subjectivity   16–18
  radical   113, 124, 130, 131
Superhealth Basic   189–90
Superhealth programmes
  182–93
  relationship to PCHP   193–5
surveys
  needs assessment   142–3
  outcome evaluation   156–7
systems   135–6
systems thinking   27

Taoistic change   122–3

targeting 31, 133
team learning 27
transpersonal/transpersonal
    experiences 111–15
    definitions 111–13
    power and 118–19
Treaty of Waitangi (1840) 105–6

unemployment, Other Way
    Project 203–13
United States
    *Healthy people: The Surgeon General's
    report* (1979) 5
    Objectives for the Nation 5
unity, community 33–4

Unstress programme 186–9

values
    definition 217
    hard/soft 215, 217–18
victim blaming 6

weight-control programme, Superhealth
    (Waistline) 184–6
well-being 36, 56–63
    subjective measures 40, 158–60
Workplace Health System (WHS) 27–8
World Health Organization
    definition of health 8, 56, 59
    Ottawa Charter 6

Index compiled by Anne McCarthy